Manual of
Small Animal
Ophthalmology

Manual of Small Animal Ophthalmology

Milton Wyman, D.V.M., M.S.

Diplomate
American College of Veterinary Ophthalmologists
Professor of Veterinary Clinical Sciences
The Ohio State University College of Veterinary Medicine
Professor of Ophthalmology
The Ohio State University College of Medicine
Columbus, Ohio

Churchill Livingstone
New York, Edinburgh, London, Melbourne   1986

Library of Congress Cataloging-in-Publication Data

Wyman, Milton.
 Manual of small animal ophthalmology.

 Bibliography: p.
 Includes index.
 1. Dogs—Diseases. 2. Cats—Diseases. 3. Veterinary
ophthalmology. I. Title.
SF992.E92W96   1986   636.7'08977   86-12975
ISBN 0-443-08317-7

Distributed in the United Kingdom by Churchill Livingstone,
Robert Stevenson House, 1-3 Baxter's Place, Leith Walk,
Edinburgh EH1 3AF, and by associated companies, branches,
and representatives throughout the world.

Accurate indications, adverse reactions, and dosage schedules
for drugs are provided in this book, but it is possible that they
may change. The reader is urged to review the package
information data of the manufacturers of the medications
mentioned.

Acquisitions Editor: *Gene C. Kearn*
Copy Editor: *Kamely Dahir*
Production Designer: *Jocelyn Eckstein*
Production Supervisor: *Jane Grochowski*

Printed in the United States of America

First published in 1986

I dedicate this manual with affection and grateful thanks to Jules and Lena Flock who provided encouragement, faith, and when needed most, financial support, without which I could not have obtained my professional education.

PREFACE

This manual was designed as a guide to the small animal practitioner for the identification, diagnosis, and management of common eye diseases in dogs and cats. By using the algorithm in the Appendix the practitioner is guided to the differential diagnosis. The diagnosed condition can be found in the Index, and the practitioner can then refer to the appropriate part of the book to find a concise description of the disease as well as an effective approach to the management of the problem. Additional suggested reading material is offered; this can be used to supplement the manual and serve as an aid to the practitioner for the management of the patient and to acknowledge the need for referral. Tables, charts, and photos are also included; they assist in drug selections, breed predisposition, and the photographic descriptions of the many conditions. The manufacturers and trade names of available drugs prove extremely helpful to the busy practitioner. This manual is not inclusive, but when used carefully and with discretion it provides an effective approach to identifying and managing most of the common oculopathies of small animals.

I have always encouraged my students to learn the anatomy of the eye. I believe that every time you examine an animal's eye, you should "study the anatomy." The better you know the eye, the easier it is to diagnose the condition and in turn design a medical or surgical procedure to alleviate the problem. With this concept in mind, I begin each section with the anatomy and physiology of the part. I encourage the reader to read this material. I feel confident it will be a valuable exercise.

I hope that the reader does not treat all eye diseases by a "cookbook" method, but thinks each disease through and investigates each lesion, which may be difficult to differentiate and whose incorrect therapy may be harmful if the condition is misdiagnosed. When the diagnosis is still undecided, referral is a viable alternative. Indeed, referring the patient may be a very helpful educational experience.

Milton Wyman, D.V.M., M.S.

CONTENTS

1

Examination of the Eye and Adnexa

ADNEXA

Gross examination must follow a systematic process after obtaining complete history (see Fig. A-1 in Appendix). It can be performed in room light.

I. Observe general appearance, for example
   A. Lid contour and conformation (see specific diseases for full description)
      1. Entropion
      2. Ectropion
      3. Abnormal placement of cilia
      4. Swellings
   B. Presence and character of ocular discharge
      1. Epiphora
      2. Purulent exudate
      3. Serosanguineous exudate
   C. Position of the membrana nictitans
      1. Prolapsed
      2. Everted
      3. Enlarged
   D. Position of the globe
      1. Exotropia
      2. Esotropia
      3. Exophthalmia
      4. Endophthalmia
   E. Size of the eye
      1. Anophthalmia or microphthalmia
      2. Phthisis bulbi
      3. Buphthalmia
   F. General appearance of the cornea
      1. Degree of transparency
      2. Ulceration or other changes in curvature
      3. Vascularization
      4. Pigmentation
   G. Facial symmetry
      1. Unilateral or bilateral involvement
      2. Facial hemiparesis
II. Examine the apparently normal eye when only one eye is affected.

EXAMINATION OF SPECIFIC STRUCTURES

  I. Generally little or no restraint necessary
   A. Tranquilization may affect tear production or intraocular pressure and should be avoided when possible.
   B. Tranquilization causes prolapse of the third eyelid, interfering with examination.
 II. Specific light source necessary
   A. Pen light with focal adapter (Welch Allyn)
   B. Direct ophthalmoscope and variable apertures
   C. Finhoff transluminator
   D. Biomicroscope (slit lamp)—expensive but most sophisticated
III. Magnification
   A. Optivisor
   B. Surgical loupe
   C. Biomicroscope
   D. Direct ophthalmoscope
IV. Recommended sequence of examination
   A. Gross examination and anamnesis (see Adnexa I & II—p. 1)
   B. Lids (all three)
     1. Lid margins
       a) Exudate
       b) Color
       c) Inflammation
       d) Misplaced hairs
       e) Deviated margins
       f) Growths or focal swelling on lids or their margins
         (1) Granulation tissue
         (2) Dermoids
         (3) Meibomian abscess
         (4) Chalazion
         (5) Neoplasms
       g) Defects of lid continuity and margins
         (1) Congenital—colobomata
         (2) Acquired—lacerations
     2. Palpebral surface
       a) Evert upper, lower, and third eyelids
       b) If topical anesthesia is necessary to perform eversion, perform the following first if indicated:
         (1) Culture specimens
         (2) Schirmer tear test
   C. Conjunctiva
     1. Evert all three lids to observe the fornices.
     2. Observe for signs of inflammation.

        a) Color—hyperemia, pallor
        b) Congestion
        c) Exudate
        d) Edema—chemosis
        e) Thickness
    3. Observe for abnormal growths.
    4. Observe for abnormal adhesions (symblepharon).
 D. Cornea
    1. Focal illumination is the most effective way to examine the cornea.
        a) Many light sources are suitable (see Adnexa—specific light source necessary).
        b) Magnification is necessary.
    2. Integrity of corneal epithelium
        a) Stain (see stains)
        b) Wood's light may be required to enhance fluorescence in subtle ulcers.
    3. Loss of transparency
        a) Edema
            (1) Anterior uveitis
            (2) Glaucoma
            (3) Endothelial damage
            (4) Interstitial keratitis
        b) Vascularization
            (1) Deep
            (2) Superficial
        c) Granulation or other cellular infiltration
        d) Pannus (pigmentary keratitis)
        e) Degeneration or dystrophy
        f) Neoplasm
 E. Sclera
    1. Inflammatory diseases
        a) Episcleritis
        b) Scleritis
    2. Discoloration
        a) Melanosis
        b) Icterus
    3. Trauma
        a) Tears
        b) Lacerations
    4. Growths and enlargements
        a) Neoplasia
        b) Granulation
 F. Anterior chamber—focal illumination necessary
    1. Abnormal content

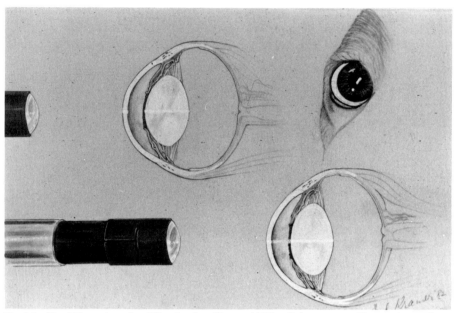

Fig. 1-1. (Top) Normal eye focal illumination. (Bottom) "Flare" demonstrated by continuous beam of light through the aqueous. Requires a focal beam to demonstrate this phenomenon.

  a) Increased protein results in "flare" (i.e., Tyndall) effect (Fig. 1-1)
  b) Anterior lens displacement
  c) Presence of cells
      (1) Hyphema—red blood cells
      (2) Hypopyon—white blood cells
      (3) Pigment—exfoliative cells from uveal epithelium or neoplasms
      (4) Keratic precipitates—debris and cells deposited on corneal endothelium
  d) Foreign bodies
  2. Depth
      a) Deep—posterior lens luxation
      b) Shallow—intumescent lens
      c) Irregular—subluxated lens—neoplasia
  3. Examine the angle—gonioscope (see Ch. 8)
G. Iris
  1. General appearance
      a) Normal
          (1) Crisp detail
          (2) Contains crypts and visible vessel pattern

　　　b) Abnormal
　　　　(1) Dull
　　　　(2) Thickened, loss of normal architecture
　　　　(3) Exudates
　　　　(4) Neovascularization
　　　　(5) Loss of substance—usually advanced
　　　　(6) Change in color—neoplastic changes or postinflammatory lesions
　　　　(7) Adhesions and inflammatory strands
　　2. Mobility
　　　a) Synechia—complete or partial immobility in involved regions
　　　　(1) Anterior—adherent to posterior surface of the cornea
　　　　(2) Posterior—adherent to anterior surface of the lens
　　　b) Mydriasis
　　　　(1) Drugs—mydriatics
　　　　(2) Oculomotor palsy—neurologic
　　　　(3) Glaucoma—fixed dilated pupil
　　　　(4) Retinal or optic nerve disease
　　　c) Miosis
　　　　(1) Drugs—miotics
　　　　(2) Iritis
　　　　(3) Sympathectomized eye—Horner's syndrome
　　　d) Pupillary response to light—not necessarily a function of vision (Fig. 1-2)
　　　　(1) Direct—pupillary response in the stimulated eye
　　　　(2) Indirect—pupillary response in the eye contralateral to the stimulated eye
　　　e) Iridodonesis—trembling of the iris with eye movement indicates loss of lens support
　　3. Atrophy—lacks thickness, may have holes visible
　　　a) Senile—seen frequently in poodles (Fig. 1-3)
　　　b) Essential
　　　　(1) Spontaneous atrophy in younger animals
　　　　(2) Idiopathic
　　　c) Some believe this causes decreased response to light—I do not—pupillary response appears adequate in most of these patients (Fig. 1-3)
H. Lens
　　1. Transparency—best identified by focal illumination
　　　a) Lenticular sclerosis—normal aging change
　　　b) Cataract—pathologic opacity of lens
　　2. Size
　　　a) Microphakia most frequent congenital lesion
　　　b) Increased size due to water uptake—intumescence

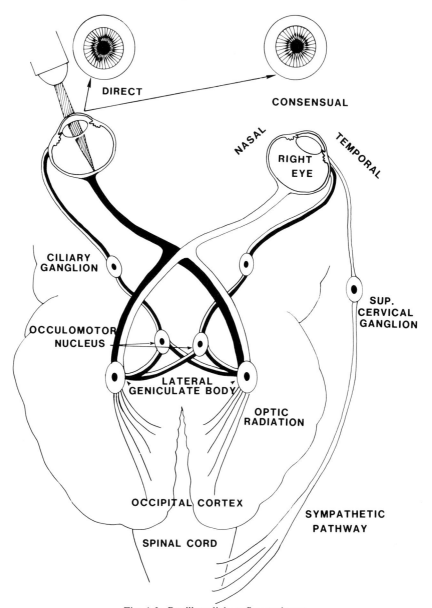

Fig. 1-2. Pupillary light reflex pathway.

3. Dislocations—subluxation or luxation; observe for aphakic crescent
   a) Direct a light into pupil 18 to 24 inches from the patient.
   b) Observe the difference of the tapetal reflection at the lens equator and the portion of which does not traverse the pupil (Fig. 1-4).

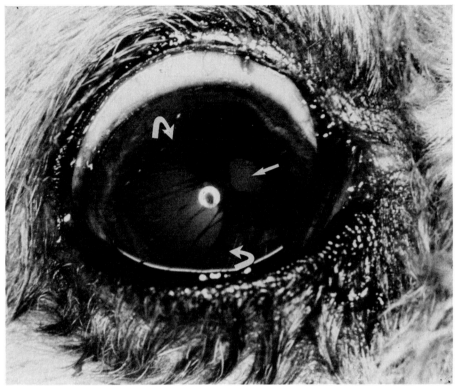

Fig. 1-3. Aged miniature poodle with clinically normal vision and senile iris atrophy. Constricted pupil (straight arrow); iridal atrophy (bent arrows).

    I. Vitreous—best examined by indirect illumination
       1. Transparency
          a) Cells—hemorrhage or exudate
          b) Persistent hyaloid or inflammatory strands
          c) Asteroid hyalosis
       2. Viscosity—syneresis (liquefaction)
    J. Retina (see Ophthalmoscopy)

OPHTHALMOSCOPY

  I. Types of ophthalmoscopes
    A. Indirect binocular (sophisticated instrument)
       1. Advantages
          a) Stereoscopic vision
          b) Large field
          c) Greater distance from patient to observer

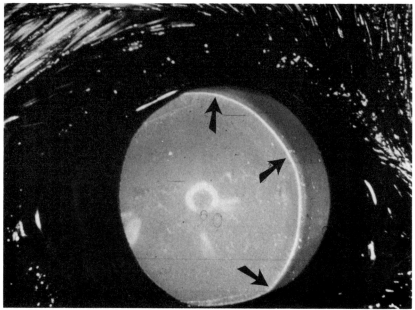

Fig. 1-4. Siberian Husky. Primary glaucoma with secondary lens subluxation. Arrows identify the equator of the lens.

d) Easier to examine peripheral fundus
e) Greater freedom of hands allows for easier manipulation of patient
f) More intense light source provides better penetration through opaque media
2. Disadvantages
a) Cost
b) Difficult to acquire the necessary skill
c) Not as portable as direct scopes
d) Inverted and backwards image
e) More difficult to examine the anterior segment for the beginner
f) Diopter determinations cannot be made
B. Inexpensive indirect binocular
1. Advantages
a) Requires inexpensive 5× magnifying lens
b) Adequate light source
(1) Pen light
(2) Direct ophthalmoscope
c) Portable
d) Easy to use with little practice
e) Quick
f) Provides a wide field, which makes it easier to identify a lesion and its location

    2. Disadvantages
      a) Cannot penetrate moderately opaque media
      b) Image is not as distinct as in more sophisticated instrument
      c) More difficult to see stereoscopically
      d) Image inverted and backwards
  C. Indirect monocular
    1. Advantages
      a) Easiest ophthalmoscope to use
      b) Provides an erect image
      c) Provides an illuminated field five times larger than the direct field
      d) Easier to examine peripheral fundus
      e) Portable instrument available
    2. Disadvantages
      a) Cost
      b) Diopter determinations cannot be made
      c) Stereoscopic vision cannot be obtained
      d) Less magnification than direct ophthalmoscope
  D. Direct
    1. Advantages
      a) Relatively inexpensive
      b) Erect image
      c) Magnified 8 to 10 times
      d) Relatively easy to master technique
      e) Can determine diopter
    2. Disadvantages
      a) Small field—approximately 5 mm
      b) Difficult to evaluate periphery
      c) Stereoscopic vision cannot be obtained
      d) Difficult to orient lesions due to small field
      e) Tendency for the examiner to accommodate to the patient's eye is difficult to overcome
II. Definitive examination
  A. Determine pupillary response to light before producing mydriasis (Fig. 1-2)
  B. Produce mydriasis
    1. Apply 1 to 2 drops tropicamide HCl 1% bilaterally
    2. Wait 10 to 15 minutes
  C. Restraint of the patient
    1. Tranquilization prolapses the third eyelid and should be avoided whenever possible.
    2. General anesthesia is contraindicated for adequate ophthalmoscopic examination.
    3. Manual restraint is the method of choice.

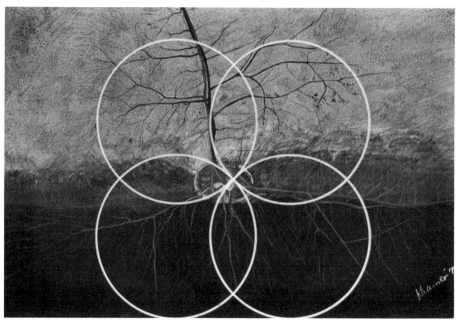

Fig. 1-5. Schematic drawing representing a cow's fundus. Overlapping circles demonstrate method of examination with direct ophthalmoscope. The examiner should direct the light into each of four quadrants using the optic disc as a reference. Allow patient's eye to move while examining each quadrant until satisfied, then move on to the next quadrant and continue until all four have been examined.

III. Use of the direct ophthalmoscope
   A. Observe patient's eye with corresponding eye of observer
   B. Hold ophthalmoscope 18 to 24 inches from patient's eye and observe the retinal reflection; examine transparent media of the eye
      1. Cornea
      2. Aqueous
      3. Lens
      4. Vitreous
   C. Follow "tapetal or retinal" reflection into the eye, bringing the ophthalmoscope within 1 to 2 inches from the patients cornea.
      1. Suppress and keep the opposite eye open.
      2. Do not accommodate to the patient's retina.
      3. Observe the retina as though looking through patient's head at a distant landscape.
      4. Eliminates observer eye strain, enabling a better examination
      5. Do not "lesion hunt"—examine the fundus in quadrants using the optic disc as a reference (Fig. 1-5).
   D. Screening examination of deeper structures
   E. Diopter settings for dogs and cats

1. Scan retina—$(-)2$ to $(+)2$ D
2. Scan vitreous—0 to $(+)8$ D
3. Scan lens—$(+)8$ to $(+)12$ D
4. Scan iris, anterior chamber, cornea—$(+)12$ to $(+)20$ D
5. The higher the positive diopter, the more difficult to examine (i.e., shorter focal length)
6. Lesions behind the equator equal 1 mm/3 D
   a) An elevated retinal lesion in focus at 6 D when the retina is in focus at 0 D extends 2 mm vitread.
   b) A cavity in the peripapillar region in focus at -6 when the retina is in focus at 0 D extends 2 mm posteriorly.
IV. Use of the indirect ophthalmoscope
   A. Place the light source and ocular prisms on the head of the observer.
   B. Adjust the interpupillary distance so that stereopsis is possible.
   C. Adjust and direct the light into the patient's eye.
   D. Place the condensing lens (various strengths) between the light source and the patient's eye, approximately 8 cm from the patient's eye.
   E. Move the lens toward and away from the patient's eye until the lens is filled with the inverse image.
   F. Use the simple indirect in much the same way, except:
      1. Hold the light source at observer's eye level and direct it into the patient's eye from 18 to 24 inches from the patient.
      2. Obtain a tapetal reflection and place the condensing lens between the light source and the reflection.
      3. Move the lens in and out, as described in part IV.E. above, to fill the entire lens area with an inverted image of the retina.

DIAGNOSTIC TECHNIQUES

I. Irrigation of the nasolacrimal drainage apparatus
   A. Equipment
      1. Nasolacrimal cannula
         a) Smooth blunted end
         b) 25- to 20-gauge cannula
            (1) Commercial
            (2) Blunt end of hypodermic needle
      2. 3- to 6-ml syringe
      3. Topical anesthetic
         a) Proparacaine 0.5%
         b) Place 1 drop in each eye; wait 5 minutes, then place another drop and wait 2 or 3 minutes.
      4. Good light source
      5. Magnification—loupe
      6. Sterile collyria

B. Technique
  1. Topically anesthetize the eye.
  2. Restrain the animal in lateral recumbent position.
  3. Tense upper lid dorsolaterally partially to evert the medial canthal area (upper puncta is my preference).
  4. Fix cannula on syringe filled with collyria.
  5. Run the cannula from lateral to medial along the mucocutaneous junction.
     a) Direct the tip slightly toward the lid.
     b) This will engage the opening and allow the cannula to enter the cannaliculi.
     c) The cannula must be parallel to the lumen or false negative patency will result.
  6. Inject collyria
     a) Watch for solution exiting the opposite punctum.
     b) Occlude the opposite punctum and inject more fluid.
     c) Exits the nose or animal coughs, gags, or sneezes as fluid enters posterior pharynx.
C. Retrograde irrigation is possible—animal must be anesthetized and nares dilated with nasal speculum to visualize meatus (see Suggested Readings)
D. Fluorescein passage technique
  1. Place concentrated dye, as in corneal staining, in the interpalpebral space.
  2. Allow 5 to 10 minutes.
  3. Observe external nares for presence of stain.
  4. This test may be negative in 30% of the test animals due to anatomy of the duct (see p. 135—Anatomy).
  5. When positive, this test demonstrates patency of the system.
II. Staining the cornea
  A. Fluorescein
    1. Used to identify defects in the corneal epithelium and stroma
    2. Must be done aseptically and atraumatically
    3. Equipment
       a) Sterile fluorescein-impregnated strips
       b) Sterile collyria
       c) Paper towels
       d) Wood's light—optional
    4. Technique
       a) Carefully moisten end of strip—larger strips may be folded lengthwise to provide rigidity.
       b) Extend the patient's neck to obtain a Doll's eye and expose the dorsal conjunctiva while the upper lid is retracted.
       c) "Touch" the moistened strip to the exposed conjunctiva, *not* the cornea.

       d) Fold a paper towel and hold below lower lid.
       e) Irrigate the cornea thoroughly with warmed collyria.
       f) Observe the surface of the eye for retention of bright green dye:
          (1) Indicative of absence of epithelium
          (2) Stroma will also stain
          (3) Descemet's membrane will not stain
  B. Rose bengal—I do not recommend for the following reasons:
    1. Vital stain (i.e., it will stain necrotic or dying cells)
    2. Nonspecific (i.e., it will stain any dead cells regardless of cause)
    3. Used in human ophthalmology to diagnose early sicca
    4. Irritating

III. Assessing lacrimation (see p. 142—Schirmer tear test)

IV. Microbial cultures
  A. When cultures are indicated they should be obtained early in the examination.
  B. On first presentation a culture is usually not necessary.
    1. If lesions persist while on medication, culture specimens can be obtained.
    2. I do not recommend delaying the culture because the animal is on therapy.
    3. If antibiotics had been effective, the patient's condition would have improved.
  C. Method—topical anesthetic is contraindicated
    1. Alginate swab is preferred.
    2. If cotton is used, it should be moistened with transport media.
    3. The eye should be irrigated with sterile saline without preservative. A sterile swab may be used to clean the eye.
    4. A specimen may be obtained from any of the conjunctival surfaces. Care should be taken not to contaminate the swab by touching the periocular skin and/or hair.
    5. Specimens are streaked on blood agar and inoculated in Hank's solution or Sabouraud's media, depending on which organisms are of concern.

V. Exfoliative cytology (see Suggested Readings)
  A. Equipment
    1. Blunt spatula (Fig. 1-6)
      a) Kimura platinum spatula
      b) Flattened piece of stainless steel surgical wire—my preference
      c) BP handle without a blade
      d) Other flat dull spatulas
    2. Topical anesthetic
    3. Clean glass slides
    4. Dif-Quick stain or others commonly found in laboratory

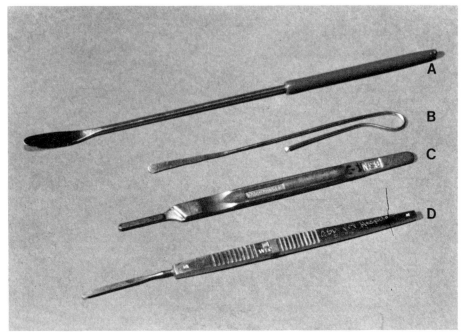

Fig. 1-6. Spatulas used to obtain specimen for cytology. (A) Inexpensive chemical spatula. (B) Stainless steel wire "home made" spatula.(C) Bard Parker #9 scalpel handle. (D) Iris repositor.

    B. Technique
       1. Anesthetize eye as in lacrimal irrigation.
       2. Evert upper or lower lid.
       3. Draw spatula across conjunctiva
         a) Move in one direction only.
         b) Elevate and draw it across again.
         c) Repeat until adequate cells are obtained.
       4. Place on clean glass slide carefully to preserve integrity of cells.
       5. Fix and stain.
 VI. Conjunctival biopsy
    A. Equipment
       1. Topical anesthetic
       2. Small Bishop–Harmon conjunctival forceps
       3. Tenotomy scissors
       4. 10% neutral formalin
    B. Technique
       1. Anesthetize the eye topically, as in lacrimal irrigation.
       2. Elevate the conjunctiva with forceps.
       3. Excise a small piece of tissue.
       4. Place in formalin and submit to the pathologist.
       5. Closing the conjunctiva is unnecessary.

VII. Tonometry (see p. 219)
VIII. Evaluating sight (see Suggested Readings)
    A. A great deal of subjectivity is innate
    B. Methods
       1. Place obstacles in the room.
       2. Ability to observe motion
          a) Swinging object
          b) Cotton balls thrown in front of patient
          c) Noiseless rolling ball or round object
       3. Menace
          a) "Threaten" animal by bringing hand close to each eye, one at a time.
          b) Do not stimulate tactile hairs.
       4. Altered light intensity
          a) Test in bright room light.
          b) Repeat in dim light.
       5. Determining visual field is extremely difficult. Careful examination may result in field deficits. For both eyes:
          a) Bring wand or suspended object into animal's nasal field (from lateral position) and evaluate response.
          b) Repeat testing of the temporal field (from medial position).
IX. Electroretinography (see Suggested Readings)
    A. Study of electrical currents produced by the retina following a light stimulus
    B. Electrodes are placed on the:
       1. Cornea or conjunctiva
       2. Posterior pole (orbital ligament)
       3. Neutral electrode (ground) on occiput
    C. Usually requires general anesthesia but can be performed in the awake animal with a computer averager
    D. Electrical potentials are recorded on an oscilliscope (Fig. 1-7)
       1. a wave—generated by rod and cones
       2. b wave—generated by the Müller cells and fibers

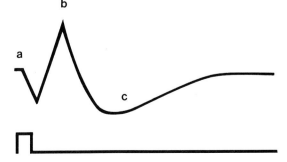

Fig. 1-7. Electroretinogram (ERG); a, b, and c waves. Bottom tracing represents light stimulus.

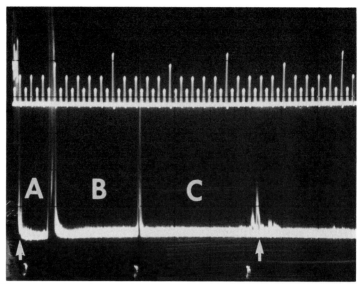

Fig. 1-8. Ultrasonography—A-scan. A, anterior chamber; B, lens; C, vitreous. Arrows indicate anterior–posterior dimensions of a normal adult dog eye.

       3. c wave—generated by RPE

   E. Used mainly to identify receptor function

   F. Of no value in identifying central, optic nerve, or ganglion cell disease

 X. Ultrasonography (see Suggested Readings)

   A. Sound waves of 500 MHz, which is above the audible range, are produced via a piezoelectrical crystal

   B. Directed through the eye, waves are obstructed by various structures to produce a recordable echo

   C. Two scans

      1. A-scan—two-dimensional echo produced by peaks of sound impedence (Fig. 1-8)

      2. B-scan—pseudo-three-dimensional echo produced by scanning through the eye; results in echo-dense areas in cross-section (Fig. 1-9)

   D. Can identify

      1. Retinal detachment when anterior segment is opaque

      2. Orbital masses

      3. Radiolucent foreign bodies

      4. Intraocular neoplasia

 XI. Fluorescein angiography

   A. Used to identify retinal and choroidal vascular disease and the integrity of the RPE or absence of normal vascular pattern

   B. When properly illuminated, intravenous or extravasated fluorescein

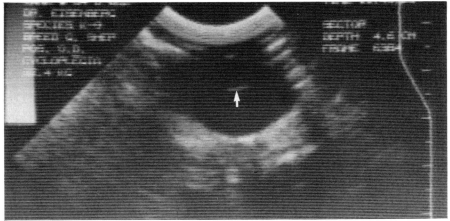

Fig. 1-9. Ultrasonography—B-scan. Small arrow represents posterior lens capsule. (Courtesy of Dr. David Herring, Section of Radiology, Ohio State University, Columbus, Ohio.)

dye will fluoresce and can be photographed or examined with special Wratton filters in the ophthalmoscope.

C. Abnormal structures will obliterate normal vascular fluorescence and can be used to outline neoplasms, etc. (Fig. 1-10).

D. Sterile fluorescein (25 mg/kg) is injected into the cephalic vein after mydriasis has been produced.

E. With the excitation filters in place, the fundus is examined in five phases:

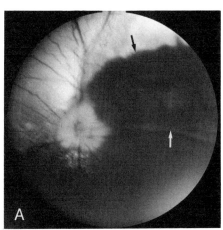
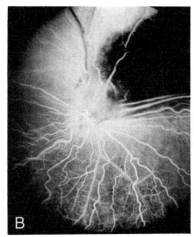

Fig. 1-10. German shepherd female 10 years old. Right eye. Presumed choroidal melanoma first observed 6 years prior to this photograph. (A) Prefluorescein demonstrating pigmented mass nasal disc. Arrows identify upper and lower limits of mass. (B) Early arterial–venous phase demonstrating avascular appearance of mass.

    1. Choroidal phase—choroidal vessels fluoresce
    2. Arterial phase—retinal arteries fluoresce
    3. Arterial–venous phase—all retinal vessels fluoresce
    4. Venous phase—some arteries and most veins fluoresce
    5. Latent phase—sclera and optic disc fluoresce for prolonged period
  F. Fluorescein "staining" results if the integrity of the vessels or RPE is compromised.
  G. This test requires proper equipment, knowledge of ocular anatomy, and experience to evaluate the results correctly.

SUGGESTED READINGS

Bistner SI: AAHA Self Study Course: Ophthalmology. American Animal Hospital Association, Denver, 1978

Blogg JR: The Eye in Veterinary Practice. 1st Ed. Vol. 1. WB Saunders, Philadelphia, 1980

Gelatt KN (ed): Veterinary Ophthalmology. 1st. Ed. Lea and Febiger, Philadelphia, 1981

Sererin GA: Veterinary Ophthalmology Notes. 2nd. Ed. College of Veterinary Medicine, Colorado State University, Fort Collins, Colorado, 1976

Slatter DH: Fundamentals of Veterinary Ophthalmology. 1st. Ed. WB Saunders, Philadelphia, 1981

2

Ocular Pharmacology

Effective treatment of disease in general and ocular disease in particular requires medication delivery to affected tissue by a route that results in a therapeutic concentration. Nothing can increase the rate of healing. Drugs can only provide an environment conducive to healing. The clinician must select every agent carefully for specific purposes, and medication should be stopped when indications are no longer present or if the lesions are static, if they persist, or if they become worse. The patient must be reevaluated frequently.

ROUTES OF ADMINISTRATION

I. Topical
  A. Effectiveness depends on
    1. Contact time—the longer the corneal contact, the higher the concentration within ocular tissues
      a) Ointments
        (1) Longer contact time than solutions
        (2) Refined ophthalmic ointment vehicles *don't retard healing*
        (3) Fat-soluble drugs penetrate the superificial cornea more rapidly than water-soluble drugs (see p. 20—Differential solubility)
          i) Ointments compete with the corneal epithelium for absorption of fat-soluble medications. This may be counteracted by increasing the concentration of the drug.
          ii) The quality of the ointment determines the bioavailability to the eye.
        (4) Should not be used on penetrated corneal laceration or conjunctival tears, because it predisposes them to lipid granulomas
      b) Viscous solutions
        (1) Better contact than aqueous solutions
        (2) Remain on the eye for shorter periods than ointments; more frequent applications required
      c) Aqueous solutions
        (1) Rapidly lost through the nasal lacrimal drainage apparatus— preferred agent for dacryocystitis
        (2) Must be applied frequently to obtain optimal levels
        (3) Often easier for the client to apply

    2. Drug dilution
      a) topical medication applied to a "tearing" eye is diluted more quickly than when applied to a hyposecreting eye.
      b) More than two drops of a solution overflows the lids and is less effective than when overflow does not occur.
      c) Allow 5 to 10 minutes between two different topical ocular drugs and precede with solution if both solution and ointment are given.
      d) Systemic absorption increases and topical ocular concentration decreases by local inflammation.
    3. Particulate size—the smaller the particle, the better the absorption
    4. Differential (biphasic) solubility
      a) Lipid solubility—nonionic phase—fat-soluble drugs reach high levels in the superficial cornea
      b) Water solubility—ionic phase—hydophlilic drugs penetrate the corneal stroma
      c) Lipid and water solubility—biphasic solubility
        i) The cornea is a fat–water–fat sandwich.
        ii) Drugs with biphasic solubility (e.g., atropine SO_4 1%) penetrate the intact cornea quickly.
  B. Intraocular concentration
    1. A superficial lesion does not require a high intraocular concentration.
    2. Biphasic solubility is important (see Differential solubility).
    3. Rate of removal
      a) Diffusion into circulating blood is via the scleral venous plexus.
      b) Rapid absorption is one of the reasons therapeutic levels cannot be reached in the back of the eye by topical administration.
      c) Inflammation results in more rapid systemic drug absorption.
    4. Many drugs concentrate in specific areas and are not uniformly distributed throughout the eye; for example, atropine has an affinity for iridal pigment.
 II. Subconjunctival or sub-Tenon injection
  A. Not a panacea for ocular drug administration—should be used with caution.
  B. For adequate levels of nonrepositol agents, daily or twice-daily injections are necessary.
  C. Painful and causes inflammation
  D. Vitreous drug levels are very low (ineffective).
  E. Higher concentrations of antibiotic can be obtained in ocular tissue by a periocular injection than by a much larger dose given parenterally.
III. Oral and parenteral
  A. There is no evidence to support oral administration of antibiotic in the treatment of bacterial corneal ulcers.
  B. Parenteral administration of antibiotic may augment ocular tissue levels achieved by topical administration.

C. Ocular inflammation enhances the penetration of antibiotics into ocular tissues and fluids due to breakdown of the blood aqueous and blood vitreous barriers.

D. Used for medicating posterior segment or lids.

IV. Retrobulbar injection—for regional anesthesia or contrast radiography

V. Intraocular injection

A. Used only when indicated for specific diseases

B. The wide range of undesirable effects that accompany this route of administration limit its therapeutic usefulness.

C. Air and/or balanced electrolyte solutions—reform anterior chamber after lens extraction or repair of collapsed anterior chamber

D. Can be used to produce phthisis bulbi (e.g., for absolute glaucoma)

VI. Retrograde arterial perfusion—of little clinical value

DELIVERY SYSTEMS

I. Occusert

A. Two semipermeable membranes with drug between

B. Not used in veterinary ophthalmology

II. Contact lens devices

A. Hard lenses—current research on a delivery system demonstrates an excellent potential for this device

B. Hydrophyllic lenses show a great deal of promise but are not technologically developed for widespread use.

ANESTHETICS

I. Topical anesthesia

A. Uses limited to

1. Tonometry
2. Gonioscopy
3. Exfoliative cytology
4. Irrigating nasolacrimal drainage apparatus
5. Examination of lids and conjunctiva
6. Removal of foreign bodies and sutures
7. Minor surgical procedures (e.g., removing redundant corneal epithelium)

B. *Never* used therapeutically

C. Topical effect—in general, they inhibit the regeneration of corneal epithelium

1. Piperocaine and lidocaine reportedly cause little or no retardation of corneal epithelial regeneration.

    2. Decreases mitosis
    3. Removes protective precorneal film by detergent action
    4. Impairs corneal ability to oxidize glucose and pyruvate; acetic acid accumulates
    5. Efficacy decreases with repeated applications
    6. Should not be incorporated in commonly used ophthalmic ointments or solutions

  D. Drugs
    1. Proparacaine 0.5% (Ophthetic, Allergan; Ophthaine, Squibb; Aktaine, Akorn)
      a) Excellent anesthetic—my preference
      b) Minor initial discomfort and irritation
      c) Rapid onset (10 to 15 seconds)
        (1) Must wait still longer for adequate anesthesia
        (2) Instill drops twice, with a 5-minute interval
      d) Store in refrigerator—ineffective when oxidized (brown)
    2. Others
      a) Tetracaine HCl 0.5%
      b) Butacaine SO_4 2%
      c) Benoxinate 0.4%
      d) Dyclonine HCl 0.5%
      e) Xylocaine 0.5%, 1%, 2% and 4%
      f) Sibucaine 0.5%

II. Regional anesthesia—used less in dogs and cats than in large animals
  A. Indications
    1. Produce akinesis for examination of the eye and adnexa
    2. Minor surgical procedures
  B. Technique—akinesia
    1. 3-ml syringe and 22-gauge needle required
    2. Infiltrate a small amount of anesthetic along the dorsal and ventral ridge of the zygomatic arch just lateral to the lateral canthus.
  C. Local infiltration adjacent to the lesion for excision
  D. Agents
    1. Procaine 1% to 4% (Novacain, Winthrop)
    2. Bupivacaine 0.25% to 0.75% (Marcaine, Breon)
    3. Lidocaine 1% to 2% (Xylocaine, Astra)

ANTICOLLAGENASE AGENTS

I. General
  A. Lytic reactions as a result of enzyme digestion are common (see p. 165—Collagenase ulceration).
  B. Devastating to the cornea
  C. Proteases are secreted by bacteria.

D. Collagenase
  1. Self-perpetuating destruction—released from necrotizing corneal tissue and granulocytes
  2. Will occur in the absence of infection (e.g., alkali burns)
II. Indication—whenever signs of keratomalacia are manifest
III. Agents
  A. Chelators of Ca ions
    1. N-acetylcysteine 10% and 20% (Mucomyst 10% and 20%, Mead Johnson)
    2. Na EDTA 0.15M
    3. Ca EDTA 0.15M
  B. Chelators of Zn ions
    1. Dimethylcysteine—make a 0.15-mol/L solution from capsules
    2. Penicillamine (Cuprimine, Merck Sharp & Dohme)
  C. Direct inhibitor (autologous serum, Alpha 2; macroglobulin)—obtain fresh blood from the patient

ANTIBACTERIAL AGENTS

I. General
  A. Many agents and combinations are available (Tables 2-1 and 2-2)
  B. A specific agent for the microbe is desirable.

Table 2-1.   INDIVIDUAL TOPICAL ANTIINFECTIVES

Individual Agent	Sources	Available Vehicles
Chloramphenicol	Alcon, Akorn Allergan, Parke–Davis	0.5% solution and 1% ointment
Colisitin sulfate (polymyxin E)	Professional Pharmacal	0.012% solution
Gentamycin*	Schering, Allergan	0.3% solution 0.3% ointment
Sulfa		
Sulfacetamide Na	Alcon, Allergan Schering, Cooper Vision,	10%, 15%, 30% solution 10% ointment
Sulfisoxazole diolamine	Roche	4% solution 4% ointment
Tetracycline	Lederle	1% solution 1% ointment
Tobramycin†	Alcon	0.3% solution 0.3% ointment
Bacitracin	Lilly, Upjohn	500 U/g ointment
Chlortetracycline	Lederle	1% ointment
Erythromycin	Dista	0.5% ointment
Neomycin	Upjohn	0.35% ointment

* Preferable drugs for *Pseudomonas*.
† Excellent for *Pseudomonas* but expensive.

Table 2-2. COMBINATIONS OF TOPICAL ANTIINFECTIVES

Combination of Agents	Sources	Available Vehicles
Neomycin sulfate, polymyxin B sulfate	Alcon, Allergan	Solution and ointments
Neomycin sulfate*, polymyxin B sulfate, gramacidin	Burroughs Wellcome, Dow, Pharmafair	Solution
Neomycin sulfate*, polymyxin B sulfate, bacitracin	Upjohn, Dow, Allergan, Burroughs Wellcome	Ointment
Oxytetracycline HCl, polymyxin B	Pfizer	Ointment

* Preferable drug for spectrum without culture sensitivity.

       1. Requires culture/sensitivity
       2. Often the antibiotic must be selected before sensitivity test results are available; use a broad-spectrum antibiotic or combination.
   C. Select topical agents that are not routinely used systemically, when possible.
   D. Prophylactic medication for elected intraocular surgery
       1. Used in preparation for an intraocular procedure
       2. I do not routinely treat prophylactically
          a) In the presence of overt signs of ocular infection, treatment prior to surgery is prudent.
          b) The patient should be treated before surgery with the specific agent until culture results are negative and clinical improvement is apparent.
   E. Spectrum—because both gram-positive and gram-negative organisms are common flora on normal dog and cat eyes, the selected antibiotic(s) should be:
       1. Effective against *Pseudomonas* and *Proteus*
       2. Effective against *Staphylococcus* and *Streptococcus*
II. Agents (Tables 2-1, 2-2, and 2-3)

ANTIMYCOTIC AGENTS

  I. Polyene antibiotics
   A. Isolated from *Streptomyces* spp
   B. Bind to sterols of sensitive fungal cell membranes to produce lethal imbalances of cell components
   C. Broad fungistatic activity
   D. Patient toxicity relates to binding to sterol moiety of renal tubular cells and erythrocytes

Table 2-3. SUSCEPTIBILITY OF COMMON OCULAR PATHOGENS TO ANTIBIOTICS

	Ampicillin	Chloramphenical	Bacitracin	Carbanicillin	Cephalosporin	Gentamycin	Tobramycin	Methicillin	Nafcillin	Neomycin	Colistin	Polymyxin B	Penicillin G	Vancomycin	Tetracycline	Sulfonamides	Kanomycin	Erythromycin
Gram-positive cocci																		
Staphylococcus (Pen-S)	S	S	S	S	S	S	S	S	S	S	R	R	S	S	S	V	V	S
Staphylococcus (Pen-R)	R	S	S	R	S	S	S	S	S	V	R	R	R	S	V	V	V	S
Streptococcus spp (B)	S	S	S	S	S	V	R	S	S	R	R	R	S	S	R	V	R	S
Gram-positive rods																		
Corynebacterium spp	S	S	S	S	S	S	S	S	S	S	S	S	S	S	S	S	S	S
Gram-negative rods																		
Pseudomonas spp	R	V	R	S	R	S	S	R	R	R	S	S	R	R	R	R	R	R
E. coli	V	V	R	S	V	S	S	R	R	V	S	S	R	R	V	V	V	R
Proteus spp	S	V	R	S	V	S	S	R	R	V	R	R	R	R	S	R	V	R
Hemophillis spp	V	S	R	S	V	S	S	R	R	S	S	S	V	R	S	R	R	V
Enterobacter	R	V	R	R	R	S	S	R	R	S	V	V	R	R	R	R	R	R
Moraxella	S	S	R	S	S	V	V	S	S	S	S	S	S	S	S	S	S	S
Chlamydia	R	S	R	R	R	R	S	R	R	R	R	R	R	R	S	S	V	R
Mycoplasma spp.	R	S	R	R	R	R	S	S	R	S	R	R	R	R	S	R	V	S

Sensitivity studies: S, 85% of the organisms tested were susceptible; V, >50% and <85% of the organisms tested were susceptible; R, <50% of the organisms tested were susceptible.

* Information compiled from Dr. Joseph Kowalski's data.

  E. Preparations
  1. Pimaricin (Natacyn, Alcon)
      a) Broad-spectrum—*Candida* and filamentous organisms
      b) Stable—well-tolerated
      c) Expensive
  2. Amphotericin-B (Fungizone, Squibb)—no available ophthalmic preparation
      a) Active against *Aspergillus, Candida, Histoplasma* and *Mucor*; variable in vitro activity against *Fusarium*
      b) Dose-related nephrotoxicity—may not be reversible
  3. Nystatin—not effective in my experience
 II. Pyrimide—flucytosine (5-fluorocytosine—Ancobon, Roche)
  A. Activity related to deamination by susceptible fungi to fluorouracil to block thymidine synthesis
  B. Effective against *Candida* and *Cryptococcus* and some strains of *Aspergilla*, *Penicillium*, and *Cladasporium*
  C. Effective aqueous and CSF levels can be obtained by oral administration
  D. Low toxicity—kidney and bone marrow function should be monitored
  E. Dose is 100 to 200 mg/kg divided qid (250- to 500-mg capsules available)
III. Imidazole compounds
  A. Alters the cell membrane and intracellular structures and interferes with synthesis or function of respiratory enzymes
  B. Broad spectrum of activity against yeast and filamentous fungi
  C. Less toxic than polyene antibiotics
  D. Agents
  1. Miconazole (Monostat IV, Ortho)
      a) Stable, well-tolerated
      b) No ophthalmic preparation available
      c) Excellent for *Candida* and *Aspirgillosis*
      d) Systemic dose is IV 30 mg/kg/day in divided doses, not to exceed 15 mg/kg/dose
      e) Topically administer IV solution as drops—q2h to q6h
      f) Subconjunctival—0.5 ml of IV solution daily
  2. Ketaconazole (Nizoral, Janssen)
      a) Well-tolerated
          (1) Blocks synthesis of testosterone
          (2) Blocks adrenal response to adrenal coricotrophin
          (3) May result in hair loss
          (4) May potentiate concommitant liver disease
              i) First orally effective broad-spectrum antifungal drug
              ii) Must be administered long (weeks or months) after clinical signs abate
              iii) Initial response takes 2 to 3 weeks
              iv) Dose is 10 mg/kg tid; in humans the depression of tes-

tosterone and elevation of liver enzymes have promoted
medicating once daily.
  3. Clotrimazole (Lotrimin 1% dermatologic cream, Schering)
      a) Broad fungistatic activity against yeasts and filamentous
         organisms
      b) Poorly active against Fusarium
      c) Well-tolerated topically
      d) Dermatologic cream applied to the eye q2h to q6h
  4. Econozole
      a) Active against a wide range of yeasts, filamentous organisms,
         and gram-positive bacteria
      b) Not currently available in the United States
IV. Compounds of dubious antifungal value
    A. Nystatin
    B. Thimerosal
    C. Tolnaftate
V. Compounds of no value for systemic mycosis
    A. Sulfonamides
    B. Griseofulvin—most effective dermatomycotic antiinfective agent
       1. Fungistatic amounts are deposited in the keratin
       2. Dose is 50 mg/kg PO sid for 6 weeks
          a) Poorly soluble in gastric fluids
          b) Administer with fat to enhance absorption

ANTIINFLAMMATORY AGENTS

I. Steroidal agents
   A. Action
      1. Decrease exudates
      2. Decrease tissue infiltration
      3. Inhibit fibroblastic activity
      4. Inhibit collagen-forming activity—potentiate collagenase activity
      5. Retard epithelial and endothelial regeneration
      6. Reduce vascularization
      7. Decrease capillary permeability
   B. Indications
      1. All allergic ocular diseases
      2. Nonpyogenic inflammations of any ocular tissue (e.g., scleritis,
         episcleritis)
      3. Reduction of scar formation
      4. Ocular surgery
         a) Cataract surgery
         b) Glaucoma surgery
         c) Keratoplasty
   C. Contraindications

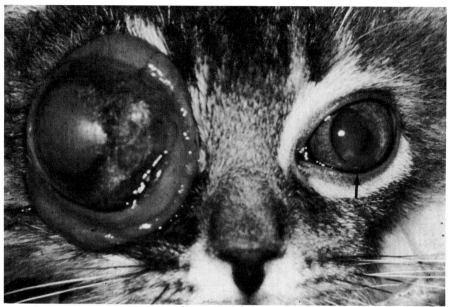

Fig. 2-1. Specific pathogen-free research kitten. Steroid-induced glaucoma and secondary exposure keratoconjunctivitis. Administered shock doses of methylprednisolone for 4 consecutive days. Protein precipitate in the left eye (arrow).

       1. Lack of specific indication for steroid use
       2. Corneal ulceration and keratomalacia
       3. Viral infections
       4. Promote fungal infection
       5. Elevate intraocular pressure in cats when given shock doses (Fig. 2-1)
       6. Predispose to cataracts in cats when used in shock doses (Fig. 2-2)
   D. Topical agents—mainly used in conjunction with antiinfective agent (Tables 2-4 and 2-5)
       1. Prednisolone acetate
          a) Acetate is lipid-soluble
          b) Penetrates epithelium well
          c) Best for superficial inflammatory diseases
       2. Dexamethasone
       3. Triamcinolone
       4. Betamethasone
   E. Systemic agents
       1. Prednisolone acetate suspension (Carter-Glogau)
          a) IM, 0.50 to 2.0 mg/kg divided tid
          b) Subconjunctivally, 25 to 50 mg, repeated 2 to 4 days later
       2. Methyl prednisolone Na succinate (Depo-Medrol, Upjohn)

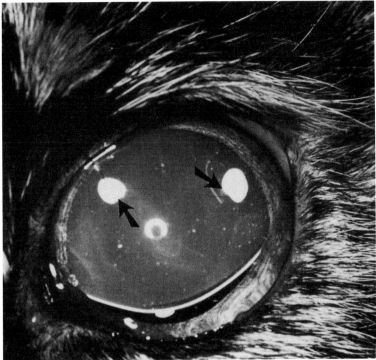

Fig. 2-2. Research cat administered immunosuppressive doses of prednisilone to facilitate *Toxoplasma* infection. Peripheral limits of sutures became opaque in approximately 80% of cats treated. Arrows identify posterior cortical opacities. Photographic artifact in the center.

   a) Subconjunctivally, 20 to 40 mg once every 2 to 4 weeks
  3. Triamcinolone (Vetalog, Squibb)
   a) IM, 0.125 to 0.2 mg/kg divided tid
   b) Subconjunctivally, 20 to 40 mg once weekly
  4. Dexamethasone (Azium, Schering)
   a) IM, 0.5 to 0.2 mg/kg divided tid
   b) Subconjunctivally, 2 to 4 mg once every week
  5. Flumethasone (Flucort, Diamond)
   a) IV or IM
      (1) Dog—0.0625 to 0.25 mg/kg/day
      (2) Cat—0.03125 to 0.125 mg/kg/day
   b) Subconjunctivally, 0.125 to 0.25 mg q48h
II. Nonsteroidal antiinflammatory agents—antiprostaglandins
  A. 20-carbon, unsaturated fatty acids
  B. Arachidonic acid and dihomo-gamma-linolenic acid are the precursors of PGE_2 and PGE_1, respectively (Fig. 2-3).
  C. Other prostaglandins are A, F, and B (Fig. 2-3)
  D. Occur in all body organs

Table 2-4. ANTIBIOTIC/STEROID COMBINATIONS: SOLUTIONS

Generic Name	Trade Name	Source
Neomycin sulfate Polymyxin B sulfate Dexamethasone 0.1%	Maxitrol AK-Trol	Alcorn Akorn
Neomycin sulfate Hydrocortisone acetate	Neo-Cortef 1.5%	Upjohn
Neomycin sulfate Polymyxin B sulfate Hydrocortisone	Cortisporin	Burroughs Wellcome
Neomycin sulfate Prednisolone	Neo-Delta-Cortef AK-Neo-Cort	Upjohn Akorn
Neomycin sulfate Presnisolone phosphate	Neo-Hydeltrasol	Merck Sharpe & Dohme
Neomycin sulfate Dexamethasone phosphate	Neo-Decadron	Merck Sharpe & Dohme
Chloramphenical Hydrocortisone acetate	Chloromycetin Hydrocortisone	Parke–Davis
Oxytetracycline HCl Hydrocortisone acetate	Terra-Cortril	Pfizer
Sulfacetamide sodium 10% Prednisolone acetate	Isopto-Cetapred AK-Cide Blephamide Metimyd Suspension	Alcon Akorn Allergan Schering

   E. Involved in
      1. Inflammation
      2. Pain
      3. Fever
      4. Smooth muscle contraction
      5. Gastric secretion
      6. Lipid and carbohydrate metabolism
      7. Cardiovascular responses
      8. Renal function
      9. Blood coagulations
   F. Endoperoxide PGG_2 and PGH_2 are pivotal in inflammation
   G. Thromboxane A_2 is essential in platelet aggregation and vasoconstriction
   H. Irin, a potent inflammatory prostaglandin first isolated from the rabbit iris, causes
      1. Severe miosis
      2. Increased vascular permiability
      3. Flare
      4. Initially, in rabbits, intraocular pressure is elevated followed within 1/2 hour by a slow decrease, resulting in hypotony

Table 2-5. ANTIBIOTIC/STEROID COMBINATIONS: OINTMENTS

Generic Name	Trade Name	Source
Neomycin sulfate Polymyxin B sulfate Dexamethasone	Maxitrol AK-Trol	Alcon Akorn
Neomycin sulfate Hydrocortisone acetate	Neocortef 0.5% Neocortef 1.5% Blephamide (0.2%)	Upjohn Allergan
Neomycin sulfate Zn bacitracin Polymyxin B sulfate Hydrocortisone	Cortisporin AK-Sporin HC	Burroughs Wellcome Akorn
Neomycin sulfate Prednisolone acetate	Neodelta-Cortef 0.5% and 0.25%	Upjohn
Neomycin sulfate Prednisolone phosphate	Neo-Hydeltrasol	Merck Sharpe & Dohme
Neomycin sulfate Methylprednisolone	Neo-Medrol	Upjohn
Chloramphenicol Polymyxin B sulfate Hydrocortisone acetate	Ophthocort	Parke–Davis
Chloramphenicol Prednisolone alcohol	Chloroptic-PSOP	Allergan
Sulfacetamide sodium Prednisolone sulfate	Cetapred AK Cide Metimyd Blephamide	Alcon Akorn Schering Allergan
Sulfacetamide sodium Prednisolone acetate Phenylephrine HCl	Vasocidin	CooperVision

I. Action
 1. Inhibit the synthesis of PGE_2 and PGF_2 alpha
 2. Prostaglandin synthesis from arachidonic acid involves many steps—antiprostaglandins suppress the activity of microsomal cyclooxygenase and arachidonic acid, inhibiting prostaglandin and thromboxane synthesis
J. Indications
 1. Before operation for intraocular surgery—administered 1/2 hour before operation
 2. Used as an adjunct to steroids or independently for anterior or posterior uveitis and endo- and panophthalmitis
 3. Focal inflammatory lesions of the lids or adnexa
K. Agents
 1. Flunixin meglumine (Banamine, Schering)
  a) Not cleared for use in small animals

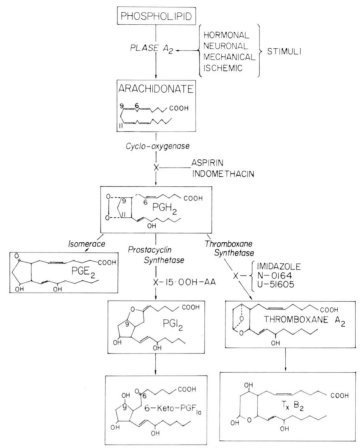

Fig. 2-3. Prostaglandin flow sheet.

b) Excellent antiprostaglandin
c) Dose—for dogs only—is 0.250 mg/kg IV only, *not* IM
2. Aspirin
    a) Excellent antiprostaglandin
    b) Dose is 1 grain per 20 pounds body weight in dogs and cats

ASTRINGENTS (LOCALLY ACTING PROTEIN PRECIPITANTS)

I. Indications
    A. Alter chronic to acute conjunctival inflammatory disease
    B. Constrict dilated blood vessels
    C. Reduce lymphoid follicle size

II. Agents
  A. Cooper sulfate crystals—should be used with caution and as a last resort, in my opinion
    1. Anesthetize the eye topically.
    2. Grasp a large crystal in a thumb forceps.
    3. Rub gently but firmly over the involved surface.
    4. Irrigate thoroughly with collyria.
  B. Zinc sulfate (Zincfrin, Alcon)—used to vasoconstrict conjunctival vessels in nonspecific, noninfectious conjunctivitis

AUTONOMIC DRUGS

I. Adrenergic action
  A. Direct-action sympathomimetic—mydriasis
    1. Epinephrine—indications
      a) Vasoconstriction
        (1) Controls capillary bleeding during surgery
        (2) Differentiates between deep and superficial conjunctival inflammation
      b) Lower intraocular pressure
        (1) Improves facility of outflow
        (2) Possibly decreases production—recent evidence challenges this theory
      c) Symptomatic therapy for Horner's syndrome
    2. Dipivalyl epinephrine (DPE) (Propine, Allergan)
      a) A prodrug
        (1) The drug is in an inactive form that is highly lipophilic and penetrates the cornea effectively and quickly.
        (2) As it penetrates. esterases break it down to epinephrine.
        (3) This results in an excellent intraocular concentration of epinephrine.
        (4) 0.1% DPE = 2% epinephrine
      b) Used for control of open-angle glaucoma
    3. Phenylephrine (neosynephrine)
      a) Mydriatic—2.5% and 10% concentrations
      b) Symptomatic therapy for Horner's syndrome
  B. Adrenergic blocking agents
    1. Beta blocker—Timolol maleate (Timoptic, Merck Sharpe & Dohme)
      a) Nonselective beta blocker
      b) Decreases intraocular pressure
        (1) Reduces aqueous formation
        (2) Increases outflow facility
        (3) Mechanism of both is unknown

c) Effective for control of occult glaucoma; not effective for acute congestive glaucoma
2. Alpha blocker—thymoxamine HCl—not commercially available
   a) Produces miosis by blocking alpha receptor of the dilator muscle
   b) Has been used in humans to treat acute narrow angle glaucoma
   c) No information in veterinary ophthalmology
C. Parasympatholytic (mydriatic/cycloplegic)
   1. Atropine—excellent mydriatic/cycloplegic
      a) One instillation may produce mydriasis lasting as long as 7 to 10 days in the normal eye.
         (1) Affinity for uveal pigment results in high concentration in heavily pigmented eyes.
         (2) Released slowly, resulting in prolonged mydriasis
         (3) Light-colored irides respond more quickly and last a shorter period.
         (4) Should not be used for routine ophthalmoscopy
      b) Blocks acetylcholine at postganlionic cholinergic nerves
      c) Absorbed readily transconjunctivally—it is not necessary to inject subconjunctivally for adequate levels
      d) May predispose to decreased lacrimal secretions
      e) Indications
         (1) Iridocyclitis
            i) Reduces pain by paralyzing the ciliary muscles
            ii) Minimizes complete posterior synechiae
               (A) Iris lens contact is less intimate when pupil is dilated
               (B) Larger pupils are less likely to become secluded
            iii) Tends to restore normal vascular permeability to the ciliary body and iris
               (A) Decreases protein and inflammatory cell concentration in the aqueous
               (B) Mechanism is unknown
         (2) Corneal abrasions
            i) Used when signs of anterior uveitis are present—only indication
            ii) Cycloplegic effect minimizes photophobia—does not stop corneal pain
         (3) Nonsurgical treatment of axial leukomas and nuclear (axial) cataracts
         (4) Attempt to free posterior synechia—1% to 4% atropine plus 10% phenylephrine
         (5) Preoperative mydriasis for cataract surgery
            i) Medicate 2 hours before operation
            ii) Use phenylephrine 10%
         (6) Postoperative cataract mydriasis

   2. Scopalamine
     a) Same action as atropine but of a much shorter duration
     b) Used in combination with phenylephrine when maximal mydriasis and cycloplegia is indicated (Murocoll-2 solution—10% phenylephrine and 0.3% Scopalamine)
     c) I do not use alone
   3. Cyclopentolate (Cyclogyl, Alcon)
     a) Primarily used for ophthalmoscopy
     b) Lasts as long as 1 to 1 1/2 days
     c) Causes severe chemosis in cocker spaniels
     d) I prefer tropicamide Hcl
   4. Tropicamide HCl (Mydriacyl, Alcon)
     a) Rapid onset—5 to 15 minutes, depending on pigmentation
     b) Short duration—5 to 6 hours
     c) Extremely safe—I have found no adverse reactions in thousands of medicated eyes
     d) May require two instillations, 5 to 10 minutes apart
   5. Oxyphenonium (Antrenyl, CIBA)
     a) Not available in an ophthalmic solution
     b) 1% solution in 1:5,000 benzalkonium chloride may be made for ophthalmic use
     c) Comparable to atropine in its action and can be used when allergy or sensitivity is associated with atropine or when atropinase is present, as in some rabbits

II. Cholinergic action—miosis and accommodation, a factor of no relative significance in veterinary ophthalmology
  A. Direct-action parasympathomimetics
   1. Acetylcholine (Miochol, CooperVision)
     a) Chemical mediator formed at
       (1) Parasympathetic nerve endings
       (2) Skeletal myoneural junctions
       (3) Ganglionic synapses
     b) Actions
       (1) Muscarinic—stimulation of postganglionic parasympathetic nerves of smooth muscle and glands
       (2) Nicotinic—stimulation of skeletal muscle and autonomic ganglia
     c) The clinical application of acetylcholine is limited to intracameral injection of 1:1,000 concentration to facilitate entrapment of anterior lens luxation during operation.
   2. Carbachol (Isopto Carbachol, Alcon)
     a) More potent and of longer duration than pilocarpine
     b) My experience with the drug on a strictly clinical basis has displayed no advantage over pilocarpine in the control of glaucoma.
     c) Combination of direct and indirect actions

   3. Pilocarpine (many available—my preference is for parasympatho-
      mimetic agents)
      a) Muscarinic actions only
         (1) Lacrimation
         (2) Salivation
         (3) Sweating
         (4) Vomiting
         (5) Diarrhea
      b) Clinical indications
         (1) Glaucoma therapy
             i) Improves facility of outflow
             ii) "Opens" closed or narrow angles
             iii) Contracts ciliary muscles improving outflow facility
         (2) Lacrimomimetic
             i) Only efficacious if some normal glandular tissue is left
                (e.g., acute daryoadenitis)
             ii) Not useful in humans, because glandular atrophy or ab-
                 sence is manifest
             iii) May stimulate production by the nictitans gland in dogs
                  and cats
             iv) I prefer topical rather than systemic use
                 (A) Less toxic
                 (B) Equally effective
                 (C) Provides tear replacement (e.g., vehicle moistens
                     the eye)
                 (D) Severin's solution (see p. 143)
      c) Available in several concentrations, from 1% to 10%
         (1) I believe 1% to 2% concentrations are the most applicable
             clinically.
         (2) Concentrations higher than 1% to 2% produce more adverse
             reactions than increased efficacy.
      d) Clients should be instructed on the adverse reactions to the drug
         initially (approximately 3 to 4 days)
         (1) Hyperemia
         (2) Protrusion of the third eyelid
         (3) Miosis
         (4) Ptosis
   B. Indirect-action
      1. Reversible—Physostigmine (eserine)—I do not use this drug
      2. Irreversible
         a) Action
            (1) Inactivates pseudocholinesterase—no direct action on mus-
                cle itself
                i) Isoflurophate (Floropryll 0.025% ointment, Merck
                   Sharpe & Dohme)

      ii) Echothiophate (Phospholine iodide 0.03%, 0.06%, 0.125%, and 0.25%—Ayerst)

    (2) Inactivates pseudocholinesterase and true cholinesterase (demecarium bromide—Humorsol 0.125% and 0.25% Merck Sharpe & Dohme)

  b) Indications

    (1) Glaucoma—as for pilocarpine, I believe there is no added benefit from these drugs and that their toxicity is too great to include them in my glaucoma regime

    (2) Treatment of parasitic blepharitis and conjunctivitis

  c) Anticholinesterase antidote Prolidoxime chloride (Protopam Chloride, Ayerst)

    (1) Action of isoflurophate, ecthiophate, and demecarium is reversed by Protopam

    (2) Administration

      i) Protopam 20 mg/kg IV slowly—may be repeated in 30 minutes using 10 mg/kg IV—must be administered within 24 hours of intoxication

      ii) Atropine should be administered—0.08 mg/kg IV every 5 to 15 minutes until symptoms regress

ANTIVIRAL

I. Action—interfere with DNA replication (herpesvirus)
  A. Replace thymidine resulting in faulty DNA production
  B. Other actions unknown
II. Indications—The only established use in veterinary medicine is the treatment of viral rhinotracheitis-induced ocular diseases of cats.
III. Agents
  A. Idoxuridine (IDU) (Herplex, Allergan; Stoxil, solution and ointment, Smith Kline & French)
  B. Vidarabine (Vira A 3% ointment, Parke–Davis)
  C. Trifluridine (Viroptic 1% solution, Burroughs Wellcome)

CAUTERANTS

I. Action
  A. Denature surface protein
  B. Effect of acid is expended, preventing deeper penetration
II. Indications—should never be used indiscriminately
  A. Sterilizes septic lesions
  B. Chemical superficial keratectomy—removes necrotic or diseased epithelium or superficial stroma

  C. Seal small "leaks" in cornea
III. Specific agents
  A. Trichloracetic acid crystals (TCA)
    1. Hydrophillic
    2. Must be kept in an air-tight vial
    3. Extremely caustic—clothing, person, and patient must be protected
    4. Applied with a small piece of cotton tightly wound around a toothpick
    5. Area touched immediately turns white
    6. Irrigate with collyria
  B. Liquid phenol (liquid carbolic acid)—similar to TCA
  C. Iodine preparations—have some anticollagenase effect
    1. 7% tincture
    2. 2 1/2% tincture
    3. Lugol's solution
    4. Xenodine

GERMICIDES

  I. Surface-active agents
  A. Benzalkonium chloride (Zephiran, Winthrop)
    1. Cationic detergent
    2. Uses
      a) Preservative for eye drops (1:5,000)
      b) Skin and eye preparation for surgery (1:5,000)
      c) Instrument disinfection (1:750)
  B. Chlorobutanol—preservative for eye drops 0.5%
 II. Sterilizing agents—ethylene oxide—excellent for sterilizing sharp instruments

INHIBITORS OF AQUEOUS SECRETION

  I. Carbonic anhydrase inhibitors
  A. Mechanism of secretory inhibition
    1. Blocks combination of carbon dioxide plus water to form carbonic acid and vice versa
    2. HCO_3 is reduced, resulting in decreased secretion
    3. Cannot completely explain reduction in IOP because of low bicarbonate ion concentration in aqueous
    4. May be due to increased hydrogen ion concentration, resulting in decreased production
  B. Not used as a diuretic per se

1. Bilateral nephrectomized rabbits had decreased intraocular pressure when administered carbonic anhydrase inhibitor
2. Used to suppress aqueous production
3. Poor diuretic in animals
   c. Agents
   1. Acetazolamide (Diamox—tablets, release capsules, and parenteral, Upjohn)—10 to 30 mg/kg divided tid
   2. Methazolamide (Nepatazane, Lederle)—4 to 8 mg/kg divided tid
   3. Dichlorphenamide (Oratrol, Alcon; Daranide, Merck Sharpe & Dohme)—2 to 5 mg/kg divided tid is my preference
   4. Ethoxzolamide (Cardrase, Upjohn)—5 to 10 mg/kg divided tid
   II. Inhibitors of sodium–potassium-activated ATP—digitalis glycosides (digoxin; digitoxin)—not used to control galucoma
   III. Sympathomimetic agents (see p. 33)
   IV. Adrenergic blocking agents (see p. 33)

OSMOTIC AGENTS

I. Mechanism of action—entirely on osmotic phenomenon
   A. Osmotic agents do not readily penetrate the blood–ocular barrier
   B. Pressure lowering is directly related to increased blood osmotic pressure
   C. Shrinks the size of the vitreous (99% water), which decreases globe content and lowers pressure
   D. Topical agents produce an osmotic gradient to withdraw fluid from cornea
II. Agents
   A. Parenteral—must withhold water
   1. Mannitol 20%—1 to 2 g/kg—slow push is my preference
   2. Glycerol anhydrous—1 to 2 g/kg PO—causes emesis in many instances
   B. Topical—for symptomatic treatment of corneal edema
   1. NaCl solutions—2% to 5%
      a) Adsorbonac (Alcon)
      b) Muro 128 (Muro)
   2. NaCl ointment (5% Muro 128, Muro)

STAINS

I. Fluorescein
   A. Water-soluble dye
   B. Turns intense green in alkaline solution
   C. Indications

    1. Stain (for identification) corneal defects
    2. Determine patency of nasolacrimal drainage system
    3. Detect small penetrating defects in cornea—produces a "fluorescein fountain"
    4. Fluorescein angiography
       a) Fluorescite 5%, 10%, and 25% (Alcon)
       b) Funduscein 10% and 25% (CooperVision)
  D. Staining mechanism
    1. Does not stain tissue per se
    2. Turns green when it contacts alkaline aqueous solution or water-soluble tissue (e.g., stroma or aqueous)
  E. Method—see Staining techniques
  F. Solutions available but not recommended because of contamination by *Pseudomonas aureginosa*
II. Rose bengal
  A. Vital dye—stains necrotic or dying cells a brilliant rose color
  B. Used in human medicine to identify early KCS
  C. Not specific—will be positive as a result of any inflammatory disease of the conjunctiva or cornea, including topical anesthesia
  D. Irritating
  E. Rose bengal sterile strips or 1% solution (Barnes–Hind; Akorn)
  F. I see no advantage to this dye in veterinary ophthalmology over more conventional diagnostic methods

TEAR REPLACEMENT AGENTS

  I. Many agents are available to supplement decreased tear production.
    A. Polyvinylpyrrolidone—my preference
      1. Similar to bovine mucin
      2. Stable
      3. Surface-wetting agent
      4. Compatible with most ophthalmic medications
    B. Polyvinyl alcohol
      1. Nontoxic
      2. Retained on the cornea slightly longer than saline
    C. Methylcellulose
      1. Viscous, water-soluble agent
      2. Nearly inert
      3. Compatible with most drugs used in ophthalmology
    D. Ethylene glycol polymers—similar to polyvinylpyrrolidone
    E. Refined petrolatum
    F. Refined lanolin
    G. Refined peanut oil
  II. Used for hyposecretion or protection the corneal surface during anesthesia

III. Agents
  A. Adapt (Alcon)
  B. Adsorbotear (Alcon)
  C. Tears Natural (Alcon)
  D. Tearisol (CooperVision)
  E. Liquifilm (Allergan)
  F. Lacri-Lube S.O.P. (Allergan)
  G. AKWA Tears ointment (Akorn)

SUGGESTED READINGS

Gelatt KN: Veterinary Ophthalmic Pharmacology and Therapeutics. 2nd. Ed. VM Publishing, Bonner Springs, KS, 1978

Havener WH: Ocular Pharmacology. 5th Ed. CV Mosby, Saint Louis, MO, 1980

Physicians' Desk Reference for Ophthalmology. 12th Ed. Medical Economics Co., Oradell, NJ, 1984

Srivivasan BD (ed): Ocular Therapeutics. Masson, New York, 1980

3
Orbit

ANATOMY AND PHYSIOLOGY

The eye of the dog and cat is contained in an incomplete bony orbit. The medial wall, from rostral to caudal, is composed of the lacrimal, palatine, frontal, and sphenoid bones. The lateral aspect is composed of the zygomatic (malar) bone. The dorsolateral aspect of the orbit is comprised of a dense collagenous orbital ligament (supraorbital ligament), which extends from the zygomatic process of the frontal bone to the frontal process of the zygomatic (malar) bone. This characteristic is, in part, a predisposing factor to traumatic proptosis in these animals. The floor of the orbit is also incomplete and predisposes to foreign body penetration per os. This incomplete cavity, then, is the scaffold that holds the eye in its functional position(s). Nerves, blood vessels, and lacrimal ducts enter and exit the orbit via foramina and fissures (Figs. 3-1 and 3-2).

The position of the eye varies with skull type, thus binocular vision, depth perception, and predisposition to proptosis are determined by conformation (Fig. 3-3). The brachycephalic dog and cat have a shallow orbit and a more anteriorly placed eye, which provides better binocular vision but a greater predisposition to proptosis. The mesatocephalic skull provides a more lateral position of the eye, thus less binocular vision but a wider field of vision. It also has a deeper orbit, which decreases the possibility of proptosis. Finally, the dolichocephalic skull type has an extreme laterally positioned eye that is deeply set in the orbit. These animals have poor binocular fields of vision and rarely present for proptosis.

The eye and all other orbital structures are invested in a connective tissue sheath, the periorbita. The periorbita lines the bones of the orbit and is adherent to the sutures. The periorbita is much thicker in those areas where bone is absent, particularly the lateral orbit. The periorbita is continuous with the periosteum of the bones of the orbital rim and the septum orbitale anteriorly.

The dura surrounding the optic nerve divides as it enters the orbit via the optic foramen, the outermost portion becoming the periorbita, and the inner portion reflected over and investing the extrinsic muscles. This inner portion is Tenon's capsule (vagina bulbi). Although oversimplified, an anology, for this structure would be the sleeve of a coat. Tenon's capsule extends to the limbus, where it is closely associated with the bulbar conjunctiva and sclera. This anatomic characteristic requires attention when preparing a conjunctival flap. When the incision is made too close to the limbus, it is impossible to exclude Tenon's capsule from the conjunctiva, which results in a very thick flap that is doomed to failure. By incising the conjunctiva approximately 2 mm posterior

43

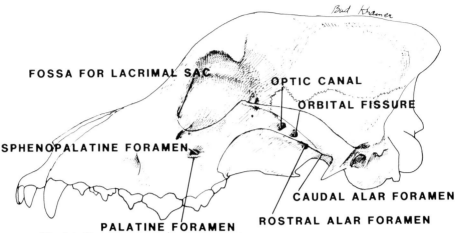

Fig. 3-1. Dog. Mesaticephalic skull type, demonstrating major orbital foramina.

to the limbus, the surgeon can easily separate Tenon's capsule from the conjunctiva, which is then more likely to remain in its transposed position.

The orbital fat pad is located between the orbital wall and the periorbita. More intraorbital fat lies between the extrinsic muscles and facial sheaths. In addition to the fat within the orbit, there are also the levator palpebrae superiorus and the seven extrinsic muscles: (1) superior (dorsal) rectus; (2) medial rectus; (3) inferior (ventral) rectus; (4) lateral rectus; (5) superior (dorsal) oblique; (6) inferior (ventral) oblique; and (7) retractor bulbi (oculi). The extrinsic muscles, except the inferior oblique muscle, originate from around the optic foramen and orbital fissure, referred to as the Annulus of Zinn. The inferior oblique originates from the medial wall of the orbit in the area of the lacrimal fossa. The anterior insertion of the medial rectus and the arrangement

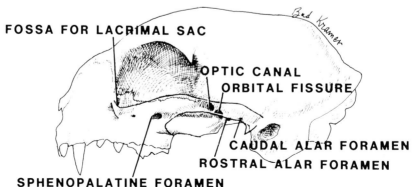

Fig. 3-2. Cat skull, demonstrating major orbital foramina.

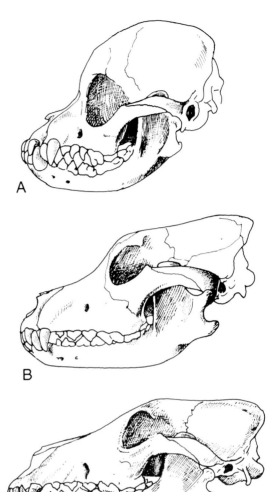

Fig. 3-3. (A) Brachycephalic. (B) Mesaticephalic. (C) Dolichocephalic skull type.

of the inferior oblique predispose these muscles to avulsion when proptosis occurs. This results in dorsal lateral deviation of gaze subsequent to this injury.

Outside the periorbita and in contact with the pterygoid muscle is a large salivary gland (zygomatic salivary gland) in the dog and a lesser one in the cat. Superficially, it is covered by the zygomatic arch and the temporal and masseter muscles. It has four to five ducts, which empty into the oral cavity by a common duct adjacent to the last upper molar. This duct is almost as large as the parotid duct but in a more caudal position. It is important to keep this in mind when performing a parotid duct transposition.

Another noteworthy anatomic characteristic is that of the check ligaments and troclea of the extrinsic muscles. The condensations of Tenon's capsule (check ligaments) prevent overaction of the muscles. The troclea is a pulley-like structure, in the dorsomedial aspect of the orbit, through which the superior oblique muscle passes toward its insertion on the dorsolateral aspect of the globe. When performing an enucleation, the surgeon should avoid including the troclea because it represents excessive dissection.

The orbit also contains the lacrimal gland, vessels, nerves, and membrana nictitans (third eyelid) (see Ch. 6).

The eye, encased in this cone-like structure, is surrounded by some of the muscles of mastication, paranasal sinuses, teeth, zygomatic salivary gland, tongue, ramus of the mandible turbinates, and the oral cavity. Diseases that affect these structures may also affect the eye and must always be considered when evaluating orbital disease.

Enophthalmos is a recession of the eyeball due to either a loss of tissue within the orbit or a congenitally large orbit. The membrana nictitans will protrude in this situation. Some pathologic causes of enophthalmos include loss of fat or muscle, dehydration, and, in rare instances, rupture of the periorbita.

It is clear why inflammatory disease and other space-occupying lesions displace the eye. The displacement is usually in the opposite direction of the mass; for example, a lesion on the medial ventral orbital wall displaces the eye dorsal laterally, and a lesion behind the eye displaces the eye anteriorly. These displacements produce exophthalmos. Often, a space-occupying orbital lesion produces a protrusion in the oral cavity because of the incomplete bony orbital floor. The oral cavity should always be examined when exophthalmos is manifest.

Often it is important to differentiate between exophthalmos and buphthalmos. One helpful diagnostic technique uses the displacement phenomenon. The test is called "retropulsion," which means to push the globe toward the orbital apex. A space-occupying mass prevents caudal displacement. The opposite eye may be used as a control.

ORBITAL INFLAMMATION:
ABCESS OR CELLULITIS

   I. Predisposing factors in small animals (see Fig. A-1 in Appendix)
     A. Incomplete orbital rim
     B. Incomplete orbital floor
     C. Tooth root abscess; position of molar roots (especially the carnassial tooth) in relation to orbit
     D. Paranasal sinuses in relation to orbit
     E. Orbital (zygomatic) salivary gland in dogs and cats
     F. Temporal and pterygoid muscles in close proximity to the globe
  II. Causes—still speculative
     A. Extension from periorbital disease
       1. Oral foreign bodies
       2. Dental abscess

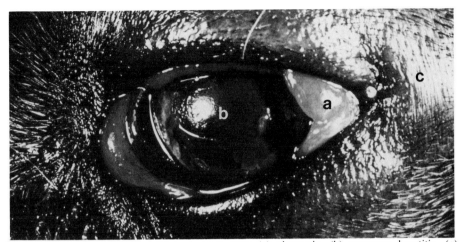

Fig. 3-4. Boxer with acute orbital abscess: note (a) chemosis, (b) exposure keratitis, (c) blepharedema.

          3. Sinusitis
          4. Cat fight (cat abscess)
          5. Zygomatic adenitis
     B. Hematogenously spread sepsis is presumed
III. Clinical signs—usually unilateral but can be bilateral
     A. Abscess (Fig. 3-4)
          1. Acute onset
          2. Pain when opening mouth—may cause anorexia
          3. Swelling of periorbital tissues
          4. Hot and painful to touch
          5. Pyrexia
          6. Swelling caudal to last upper molar
          7. Conjunctivitis and chemosis
          8. Blepharitis or blepharedema
          9. Keratitis
         10. Uvetitis
         11. Prominent third eyelid
         12. Deviation of gaze
         13. Possible blindness
     B. Cellulitis
          1. Chronic
          2. Less painful than an abcess
          3. Fever absent or minor
          4. More generalized swelling rather than pockets
IV. Diagnosis
     A. Clinical signs
     B. Diagnostic tests (p. 60)

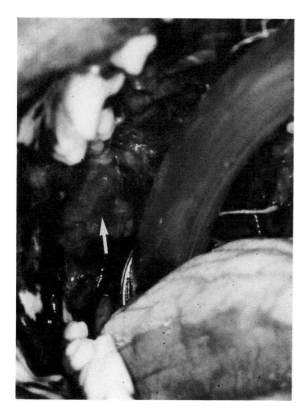

Fig. 3-5. Area posterior to last upper molar. Arrow indicates dorsal hyperemic, swollen area, indicating position to incise for drainage.

V. Treatment
   A. Establish bottom drainage
      1. Little exudate observed in cellulitis
      2. Copious amounts of exudate often observed with abscess
   B. Method
      1. General anesthesia
      2. Incise the oral mucosa immediately caudal to the last molar with a #11 BP (Fig. 3-5).
      3. Place a curved Crile hemostat in the incision.
         a) Direct toward orbit
         b) Insert closed, then open gently
      4. Exudate may or may not be observed.
      5. The procedure should not be considered inoccuous.
      6. Do not irrigate.
         a) May result in inspisation of irrigant
         b) May complicate disease
            (1) Contributes to exophthalmos
            (2) Spreads infection
   C. Extract involved teeth.

D. Administer systemic antibiotics and steroids, if necessary.
E. Medicate the eye as the clinical condition dictates (e.g., with anti-biotics, lubricants, or mydriatics).
F. Use warm compresses; if exophthalmic, use cautiously.
G. A diet of soft food is prudent.
VI. Prognosis—excellent to guarded, depending on severity, duration, and cause

ENOPHTHALMOS

I. Horner's syndrome—a sympathectomized eye. Nerve tracks originate in the hypothalamus and pass through the brainstem, cervical spinal cord, lower cervical sympathetic ganglia, vagosympathetic trunks, internal carotid plexi, and intraorbital.
A. Causes
    1. Trauma to the sympathetic trunk
    2. Neoplasia along sympathetic trunk
    3. Chronic otitis media or interna
    4. Surgery
    5. Disc disease
    6. Idiopathic—spontaneously observed, especially in collies
B. Clinical signs (Figs. 3-6 and 3-7)
    1. Ptosis
    2. Miosis
    3. Enophthalmos
    4. Prolapse of the nictitating membrane
    5. Increased heat of the pinna on the affected side—difficult to identify

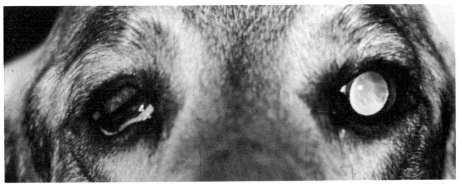

Fig. 3-6. Beagle with iatrogenically simulated Horner's syndrome produced with topical application of 1% pilocarpine solution. Right eye demonstrates typical clinical signs: ptosis, enophthalmos, miosis, and prominent third eyelid.

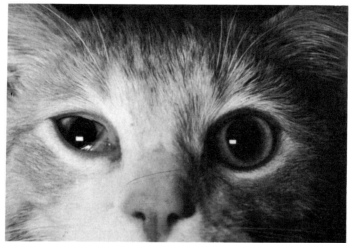

Fig. 3-7. DSH female, 2 years old, with spontaneous (transient) Horner's syndrome, right eye.

      6. Vasodilation results in a "pink" appearance of skin on affected side in white or lightly pigmented animals
      7. Very transient decrease in intraocular pressure—not clinically significant
    C. Diagnosis
      1. Clinical signs
      2. Determine location by pharmacologic tests
        a) 1% hydroxyamphetamine
          (1) First- (central) and second- (preganglionic) order neurons—normal dilation
          (2) Third-order neuron (postganglionic)—incomplete dilation
        b) 10% phenylephrine—confirmatory test
          (1) First- and second-order neurons—no dilation
          (2) Third-order neuron—normal dilation
    D. Treatment
      1. Transient disease is self-limiting. To allay client concern during recovery, symptomatic therapy may be offered—topical 2.5% phenylephrine sid or bid.
      2. Dependent on cause—primary lesion must be identified and treated if possible
    E. Prognosis—dependent on cause
      1. Simple trauma or surgery—transient, with an excellent prognosis
      2. Avulsion of brachial plexus—grave
      3. Otitis media or interna—grave
      4. Disc disease—guarded
 II. Nonspecific enophthalmos
    A. Characteristic of certain breeds (e.g., Irish setter)

           1. Associated with an enlarged orbit
           2. Predisposes to entropion (see p. 79)
    B. Loss of orbital tissue
           1. Dehydration
           2. Loss of fat
           3. Muscle atrophy
    C. Often a sign of superficial painful oculopathy
           1. Keratitis (i.e., ulcers or lacerations)
           2. Conjunctivitis, especially in cats
           3. Foreign bodies in cul-de-sacs or under membrana (third eyelid)
           4. Evaluation must include identifying the specific disease; for management, refer to the specific etiology
III. Atrophic myositis
    A. Etiology
           1. Unknown
           2. May be the sequela to recurrent eosinophillic myositis
    B. Clinical signs
           1. Atrophy of the temporal and masticatory muscles
           2. Enophthalmos
           3. Inability to open mouth
           4. Eventually, weight loss
    C. Diagnosis
           1. By observation
           2. Muscle biopsy
    D. Treatment (see Suggested Readings)
    E. Prognosis—guarded

EXOPHTHALMOS

  I. General—increase in volume of tissues within the orbit (Figs. 3-4, 3-8 and A-1)
    A. Displaces the eye
    B. Prevents retropulsion
 II. Eosinophilic myositis (Fig. 3-8)
    A. Breed predisposition
           1. German shepherds
           2. Weimaraners
           3. Has rarely been diagnosed in other breeds
    B. Etiology—unclear, but may be:
           1. Autoimmune disease
           2. Allergy
    C. Clinical signs
           1. Usually bilateral masticatory muscle swelling
           2. Pain on opening the mouth—trismus

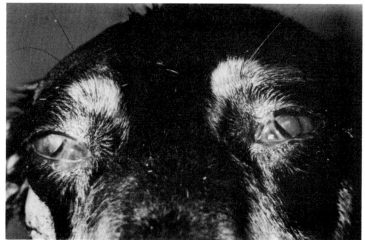

Fig. 3-8. Eosinophilic myositis in a Doberman pinscher. Diagnosis confirmed by biopsy. Note the prominence of the eyes and membrana nictitans.

    3. Protrusion of the third eyelid
    4. Blepharoedema
    5. Severe exophthalmos results in:
        a) Exposure keratitis
        b) Conjunctivitis
        c) Anterior uveitis due to exposure
    6. May have intermittent swelling (1 or 2 weeks) and recovery—recurrence results in:
        a) Muscle atrophy
        b) Enophthalmos
        c) Difficulty in opening the mouth
  D. Diagnosis
    1. Clinical signs
    2. Elevated serum muscle enzymes
    3. Mild leukocytosis
    4. Variable eosinophilia
    5. Plasma proteins and beta globulins have been reported elevated
    6. Muscle biopsy—best diagnostic tool
        a) Mononuclear cell infiltrates
        b) Polymorphonuclear cell infiltrates, many of which are eosinophils
  E. Treatment—corticosteroids—prednisilone
    1. 2 to 4 mg/kg at reducing levels
    2. If exacerbation occurs, alternate days of 1/2 mg/kg or to effect.
  F. Prognosis
    1. Recurrences are common.

2. Severe acute attacks have reportedly been fatal.
3. Usually responsive to therapy with a fair to good prognosis

TRAUMATIC PROPTOSIS (Fig. 3-9)

I. Etiologies
  A. Automobile injuries or other blunt contusion
  B. Big animal–little animal confrontation
II. Clinical signs
  A. Eye displaced rostral to free lid margins—most common in prominent-eyed brachycephalic skull types
  B. Conjunctival involvement
    1. Congestion
    2. Chemosis
    3. Hemorrhage
    4. Tears
    5. Desiccation
  C. Dorsal lateral deviation of gaze (Fig. 3-10)
    1. Due to avulsion of the medial rectus and inferior oblique muscles
    2. Degree depends on the extent of injury

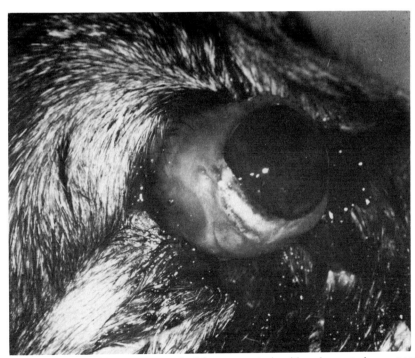

Fig. 3-9. Terrier cross with acute traumatic right eye proptosis with a clear anterior segment.

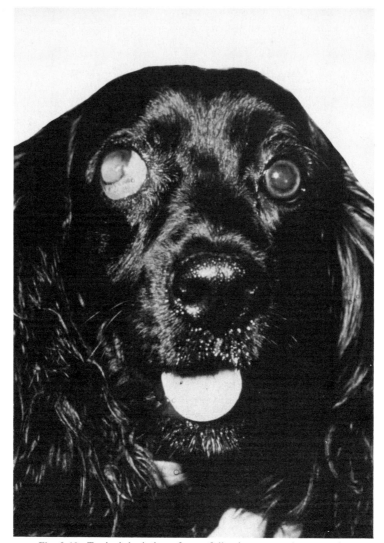

Fig. 3-10. Typical deviation of gaze following traumatic proptosis.

D. Corneal involvement
   1. Associated with degree of injury
   2. Corneal ulceration
   3. Corneal desiccation
   4. Lacerations
E. Anterior segment
   1. May be clear (Fig. 3-11)
   2. May manifest complete hyphema

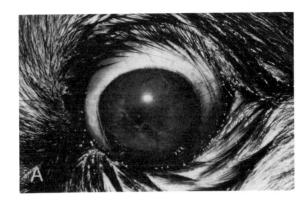

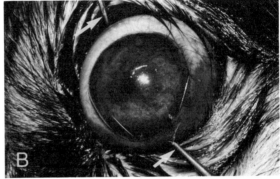

Fig. 3-11. (A) Acute proptosis. (B) Placement of muscle (strabismus) hooks to relieve lid pressure on proptosed globe (arrows). Note clear anterior segment. (C) After replacement.

      3. May manifest severe anterior uveitis
   F. Posterior segment
      1. Vitreal retinal and/or choroidal hemorrhage
      2. Retinal detachment
      3. Retinal tears
   G. Optic nerve
      1. Avulsion

      2. Hemorrhage

      3. Inflammation

      4. Chronic lesions result in atrophy

III. Diagnosis—clinical signs

IV. Treatment

    A. Evaluate and treat the patient for shock and other critical injuries or abnormalities.

    B. Induce general anesthesia.

    C. Gently cleanse the globe and lids.

      1. Gently and thoroughly irrigate with warmed saline.

      2. Fluid-soaked cotton, rather than a gauze pad, is preferred for cleansing the eye.

      3. Hypertonic solutions are contraindicated, in my opinion.

      4. Avoid lipid ointments.

      5. Water-soluble solutions are preferred as a lubricant.

    D. The objective is to free the entrapped globe from in front of the lids:

      1. Use two strabismus hooks.

        a) Engage the upper and lower lid with the hooks.

        b) Apply gentle pressure out and away from the entrapped globe (Fig. 3-11B).

        c) The eye will return to its normal position unless:

          (1) Orbital hemorrhage is excessive

          (2) Orbital edema is excessive

          (3) Muscle avulsion is excessive

      2. Alternate method (Severin's technique)

        a) Place three sutures into the lids, as for a tarsorrhaphy (Fig. 3-12).

        b) Place a scalpel handle between the eye and the preplaced sutures.

        c) Apply tension to the sutures.

        d) This results in globe replacement.

        e) Tie the sutures.

      3. Relief of the lid stricture will:

        a) Reestablish blood flow

        b) Reestablish lymph flow

        c) Minimize edema, swelling, and corneal irritation

      4. Temporary tarsorrhaphies are indicated in severe proptosis resulting in lagophthalmos, but not for simple, uncomplicated proptosis.

      5. Some ophthalmologists advocate injecting steroids retrobulbarly—*I do not*

        a) The compromised orbit does not need further insult.

        b) If steroids are indicated, use them systemically.

      6. Systemic antibiotics

        a) Broad-spectrum (prophylacticly)

        b) Ampicillin—20 mg/kg tid for 7 to 10 days is my preference

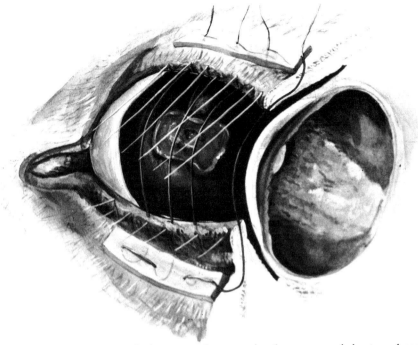

Fig. 3-12. Schematic drawing of a horse eye, demonstrating the recommended suture placement for temporary tarsorrphaphy.

       7. Topical antibiotics if there is a corneal injury
         a) Can be inserted at the medial canthus if temporary tarsorrhaphy is necessary
         b) Give tid, or more frequently if necessary
       8. Topical atropine SO_4 1% bid or tid if there is evidence of anterior uveitis
  V. Sequela to proptosis
     A. Blindness due to optic nerve or vascular injuries is common
     B. Phthisis bulbi
     C. Deviation of gaze (Fig. 3-10)
       1. Management
         a) Wait for the eye to return to normal position
           (1) May never return to normal
           (2) May require a permanent medial tarsorrhaphy to prevent exposure keratitis
         b) Muscle surgery—my preference
           (1) Complex
           (2) Should be referred to specialist
     D. Temporary or permanent orbicularis palsy
  VI. Prognosis

A. Sight—grave
B. Cosmesis—good to fair

ORBITAL FRACTURES

  I. Less common in small animals than in horses
 II. Etiology—trauma
III. Clinical signs
    A. Distortion of the periorbital region
    B. Epistaxis
    C. Deviation of gaze
    D. Blepharoedema
    E. Chemosis and conjunctival injection
IV. Diagnosis
    A. Clinical signs
    B. Radiographs
       1. Use normal side for comparison.
       2. Use radiopaque markers on the lid for orientation.
       3. Two views are essential.
  V. Treatment
    A. Open reduction is the method of choice.
    B. Make an adequate incision over the zygomatic arch.
    C. Bluntly dissect to the fracture.
    D. Manipulate the tissues gently.
    E. Reduction usually can be accomplished with an elevator or bone forceps.
    F. Fixation and alignment
       1. Wiring
          a) Drill two holes in each fragment with a bone pin and chuck to accomodate an 18-gauge steel suture.
          b) Form a figure-of-eight wire suture pattern using the preplaced holes.
          c) Tighten securely.
       2. Plating can be performed using small finger plates and screws.
VI. Prognosis—excellent for vision and cosmesis

ORBITAL NEOPLASIA

  I. Primary neoplasms may arise from any tissue type contained within the orbit (e.g., muscle, fascia, nerve, cartilage, gland, fat, blood vessels, lymphatic tissue, and/or bone).
 II. Secondary neoplasms
    A. Usually there is invasion from periorbital structures.

1. Oral cavity
2. Paranasal sinuses
3. Bone
        B. Rarely, there is invasion from distant sites.
III. Clinical signs
        A. Deviation of gaze—direction of deviation identifies position of mass
            1. Dorsal lateral displacement—mass medial ventral
            2. Exophthalmos—posterior or apex of the orbit
        B. Usually incidious clinical course—rarely acute
        C. Orbital deformity
        D. Progressive exophthalmos—globe will not retropulse
            1. Gently press on globe over closed eyelids
            2. Will not retropulse with a space-occupying mass
        E. Protrusion of the third eyelid
        F. Blepharitis and edema
        G. Conjunctivitis and chemosis
        H. Exposure keratitis
        I. Variable degrees of uveitis—secondary lesions associated with exposure
        J. Ophthalmoscopic lesions
            1. Localized lesions may produce elevations in the retina that appear to "move" when the globe moves (Fig. 3-13).
            2. May appear as striate
        K. Ocular immobility is a late secondary lesion
 IV. Diagnosis

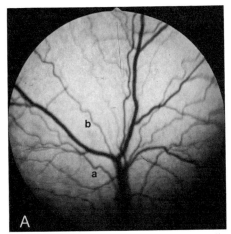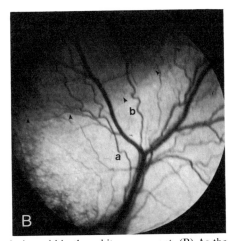

Fig. 3-13. (A) Cocker spaniel, fundus. A solitary lesion within the orbit was present. (B) As the eye moved, the lesion appeared to move. Compare A and B. The mass was depressing the fibrous tunic and changed the relative ophthalmoscopic appearance as the eye moved. Small arrows outline mass; a and b identify the same vessel in each photo. Pictures were taken on the same day and at the same time.

A. Complete history and ocular examination
B. Clinical signs
C. Sophisticated diagnostic tests
   1. Aspiration
      a) Anesthetize or heavily sedate the animal.
      b) Introduce a 2.5-cm, 20-gauge needle attached to a 3-ml syringe.
         (1) Adjacent and medial to the third eyelid
         (2) Point close to medial orbit
         (3) Aspiriate gently
         (4) Prepare specimen for:
            i) Cytologic study
            ii) Culture
      c) Alternative approach
         (1) Ocular deviation may dictate other sites of needle insertion.
         (2) A review of the anatomy would be prudent.
      d) May be used to identify:
         (1) Abscess formation
         (2) Zygomatic mucocele
         (3) Orbital neoplasia
   2. Contrast angiography
      a) Orbital venography
         (1) Inject 5 to 6 ml of Hypaque (Winthrop) or other suitable contrast medium into the angularis oculi vein.
         (2) Expose the film during injection.
         (3) Perform the technique on the opposite eye for a normal comparison.
         (4) See Suggested Readings for specific technique.
      b) Contrast arteriography
         (1) Inject the infraorbital artery with contrast media.
         (2) Limited practical application in general practice
   3. Contrast orbitography
      a) Contrast material injected retrobulbarly
         (1) Air
         (2) Opaque IV contrast material
      b) Identifies:
         (1) Radiolucent foreign objects
         (2) Space-occupying orbital masses
      c) Technique described by Barth is my method of choice (see Suggested Readings)
   4. Orbital ultrasonography
      a) Relatively new—available in large practices and institutions
      b) Useful and will be more commonplace in the future
V. Treatment
  A. Depends on type and extent of neoplasm

B. Modalities of treatment are similar to those used for neoplastic diseases elsewhere in the body
   1. Surgical and excision—method depends on site and extent of neoplasm
      a) Benign—excisional biopsy if possible
      b) Exenterate the orbit if diffuse
   2. Chemotherapy (see Suggested Readings)
   3. Radiation therapy (see Suggested Readings)
   4. Immunotherapy (see Suggested Readings)

SUGGESTED READINGS

Duncan ID, Griffiths IR: Inflammatory muscle disease in the dog. In: Kirk (ed): Current Veterinary Therapy. Vol. 7. Small Animal Practice. WB Saunders, Philadelphia, 1980

Munger RJ, Ackerman N: Retrobulbar injections to the dog: a comparison of three techniques. JAAHA 14:490, 1978

Theilen GH, Madewell BR: Veterinary Cancer Medicine. 1st Ed. Lea and Febiger, Philadelphia, 1979

4

The Eyelids

ANATOMY AND PHYSIOLOGY

The eyelids are modified integumental folds of a more delicate nature than skin elsewhere on the body. Cats, especially tomcats, however, have thicker eyelid skin than dogs.

A simplified approach to the anatomy and physiology of the eyelids is to consider that they function to: 1) protect the eye from trauma and foreign material; 2) secrete portions of the precorneal tear film; 3) spread the precorneal tear film; 4) provide a "pumping" action to propel tears to the lacrimal lake during blinking; 5) provide the entrance to the lacrimal drainage apparatus; and 6) prevent light from entering the eye.

Protecting the Eye

Tactile hairs (cilia) are found on the upper lids in dogs. On histologic and gross examination, cilia can be demonstrated in cats, but they are less distinct than in dogs. Cilia stimulation results in a protective blink reflex. They are innervated by branches of the fifth cranial nerve. Large tactile hairs (vibrissae) found around the eyes and face of domestic animals, also are innervated by branches of the fifth nerve. Vibrissae are sensitive to air currents and touch; when stimulated, they illicit a blink. When the "menace" reflex is evaluated, care should be taken not to stimulate blinking by air currents or touch.

The corneal and conjunctival surfaces are also richly endowed with sensory nerve endings of the fifth cranial nerve. Stimulation of these structures illicits a blink as well as lacrimation. Both reactions are protective to the delicate structures of the eye.

Motor innervation for eyelid closure is the auricular palpebral branch of the seventh cranial nerve. The major "sphincter" is the orbicularis oculi muscle, which encircles the palpebral fissure restricted by the medial canthal ligament and the lateral retractor anguli oculi muscle (Fig. 4-1). The latter, in animals, takes the place of the lateral canthal ligament in humans. Eyelid closure progresses from lateral to medial in a zipper-like fashion, propelling tears to the lacrimal lake (listed as the fourth function above). Phase photography demonstrates this phenomenon.

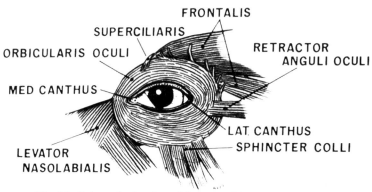

Fig. 4-1. Schematic drawing of the major lid muscles in the dog.

Secreting Portions of the Tear Film

There are two components of lacrimal secretions; basic tear and reflex tear secretions. Tear secretion is a very complex physiologic function. This discussion, although oversimplified, is important for understanding the clinical diseases associated with abnormal lacrimal function. There is an integral relationship between the tear-forming glands and the lids.

Basic Tears

Basic tear secretions contain protein (mucin), water (serous), and fat (lipid), respectively, from the epithelial surface out. The epithelium itself is hydrophobic, and something must increase its wettability to keep it moist and optically clear. This is accomplished by mucin, which interdigitates with the microvilli of the superficial epithelial cells. Mucin is produced by intraepithelial conjunctival "goblet cells," most plentiful in the fornix. These cells proliferate in chronic conjunctival irritation, giving a thickened, velvety appearance to the conjunctiva and producing increased quantity of mucin that is grossly visible.

The second (middle) portion of the precorneal film is serous, secreted by the lacrimal and nictitan glands and probably other accessory lacrimal glands as well. The accessory glands of Krause and Wolfring are commonly found in humans; however, more basic research is necessary to identify their presence in animals. The glands mentioned are considered the origin of the serous portion of the precorneal film. Secretion from the accessory glands takes place normally, without stimulation.

The outermost layer of the precorneal film is lipid secreted by the tarsal (meibomian) glands, and possibly the glands of Zeis, sebaceous glands at the base of the follicle. The lipid layer prevents overflow of tears by increasing the tear surface tension at the lid interface.

The functions of the precorneal film are to lubricate the lids as they move over the cornea and conjunctiva to provide a medium for oxygen transfer to the cornea, a vehicle for transport of antibodies and inflammatory cells to the corneal surface, an optically smooth surface on the cornea (as in polishing an optical lens), and movement of foreign material from the surface of the eye.

Reflex Tears

Reflex tears are produced by the lacrimal and nictitan glands in response to corneal, conjunctival, and lid irritation or stimulation. Humans also produce tears in response to psychic and olfactory stimuli. The afferent path for reflex tearing is the ophthalmic branch of the fifth (trigeminal) nerve to the brain stem. The efferent pathway in animals is not well understood, but branches of the facial nerve, carrying both parasympathetic and sympathetic fibers, have been traced to both glands. The clinical response to lacrimomimetic drugs, such as pilocarpine, supports the hypothesis of the parasympathetic innervation of lacrimal secretion.

Spreading the Precorneal Film

The lids, including the third eyelid, spread the precorneal film across the corneal and conjunctival surfaces. Absence of or incomplete blinking (lagophthalmus) causes drying of the corneal surface, resulting in secondary exposure keratitis. In addition, the surface imperfections of the cornea are accentuated; thus vision is impaired. Impairment of oxygen, cell, and antibody transport contributes to secondary keratitis. There has been no definitive research to determine the number of blinks per unit time in domestic animals, but the eyelids move across the eye frequently to spread tears and propel them to the lacrimal lake, located in the medial canthus.

Providing "Pumping" Action

The pumping action is integral to spreading the precorneal film. Lid closure is lateral to medial, propelling tears medially during the blink. The openings of the nasolacrimal drainage apparatus (puncta) are located at the upper and lower mucocutaneous junction, close to the medial canthus (Fig. 4-2). The puncta continue as the upper and lower canaliculi and join beneath the medial canthal ligament as the lacrimal sac. The blink propels tears medially and evacuates the accumulated tears from the canaliculi into the lacrimal sac, which dilates during the blink to produce negative pressure within its lumen. When the eyelids relax, the canaliculi dilate, resulting in negative pressure within their lumen. The lacrimal sac is compressed, evacuating the tears into the

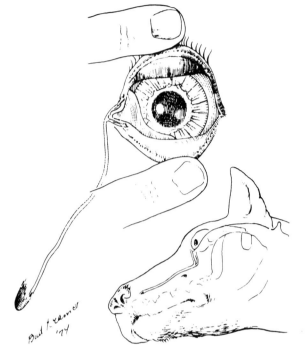

Fig. 4-2. Schematic drawing of the lacrimal drainage apparatus in the dog.

nasolacrimal ducts. Thus the blink is also necessary for normal tear removal from the interpalpebral space. Evaporation of tears from the surface of the eye is approximately 25%.

Providing Beginning of the Lacrimal Drainage Apparatus

The lacrimal puncta are in the medial canthal area at the mucocutaneous junction, close to the nasal termination of the tarsal glands. In contrast to humans, whose puncta are elevated, dogs and cats have slit-like puncta. In the pigmented conjunctiva, this structure appears as an elongated pink slit. The puncta are continued as delicate tubules, called canaliculi (see p. 65) (Fig. 4-3). The canaliculi lie close to the conjunctival surface and course medially to join underneath the medial palpebral ligament. Their junction is the lacrimal sac, which is poorly developed compared with that in primates. The lacrimal sac lies in the lacrimal fossa of the lacrimal bone, then continues as the nasolacrimal duct through the lacrimal canal of the lacrimal bone. The remaining portions of the duct course in soft tissue. The duct often has defects between the end of the lacrimal canal and the root of the canine tooth. During irrigation of the duct, the patient may cough or sneeze but have no fluid escape from the nares. The fluid enters the oral cavity or the turbinates, resulting in a gag or sneeze.

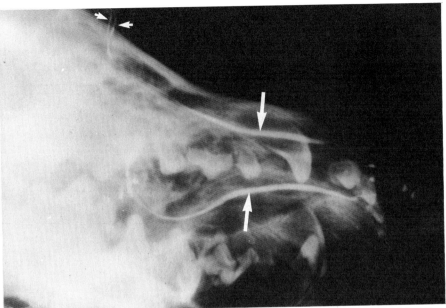

Fig. 4-3. Dacryocystorhinography of a dog's skull; canaliculi (small arrows) nasoacrimal duct (large arrows).

The distal openings of the ducts in dogs and cats are ventrolateral near the margin of the alar fold. They can be observed by dilating the nares with a speculum. If necessary, they can be cannulated for retrograde irrigation of the drainage apparatus.

Preventing Light from Entering the Eye

This function is self-explanatory, but it does have clinical implications. During sleep, the eyelids are normally closed, protecting the eye from light and dryness. Lagophthalmos may cause the patient to sleep with its eyes open. This apparently does not prevent sleep, but it does result in drying of the corneal surface, with subsequent epithelial errosion and exposure keratitis. This problem is most frequently observed in brachycephalic, prominent-eyed dogs.

INHERITED OR CONGENITAL DISEASES

I. Agenesis—absence of all or part of the lid
   A. General
      1. Has been referred to as an "atypical coloboma"

   2. Observed in the upper lateral lid of domestic cats and captive tigers
      (Fig. 4-4)
   3. Not reported in dogs in this anatomic position
      a) Defects in the ventral lid have been observed in dogs (Fig. 4-
         5)
      b) Often associated with abnormal islets of skin (see Dermoids,
         p. 70) (Fig. 4-5)
B. Etiology
   1. Unknown—congenital in cats, possibly inherited
   2. Trauma—resulting in a defect resembling a congenital lesion
C. Clinical signs
   1. Absence of the dorsal lateral lid—unilateral or bilateral (Fig. 4-4)
   2. Involves skin, tarsus, and conjunctiva to varying degrees
   3. Exposure keratitis (see p. 165—Cornea)
   4. Congenital defects identified when eyes open (10 to 14 days old)
D. Diagnosis—clinical signs
E. Treatment—requires surgery
   1. Full-thickness skin–tarso–conjunctival flap (Fig. 4-6)
      a) Form pedicle flap from the lower lid, excluding the free lid
         margin and tarsal plate.
      b) Prepare the upper lid to receive the pedicle.
      c) Pass the lower lid pedicle under the lower lid free margin.
      d) Suture together the upper cul-de-sac and lower lid pedicle with
         7-0 chromic gut.

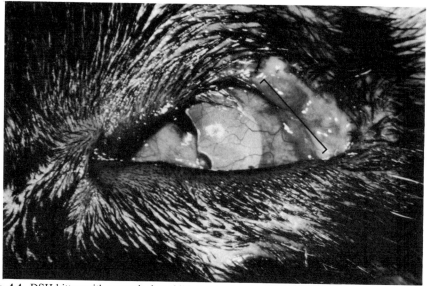

Fig. 4-4. DSH kitten with agenesis dorsal lid margin–bracket. Lesions were in both upper eyelids.

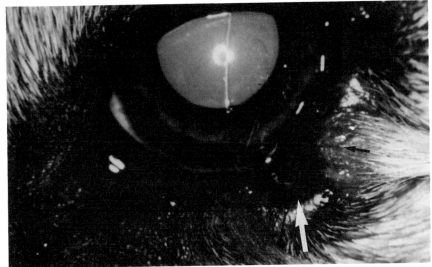

Fig. 4-5. Mixed breed 7-month old male dog with ventral lid coloboma (large white arrow) and associated dermoid (small arrow).

Fig. 4-6. Repair of upper lateral lid defect in a goat. Arrow shows the lower lid margin and tarsus. (a) Tarso conjunctival pedical from lower lid. (b) Bed in upper lid defect.

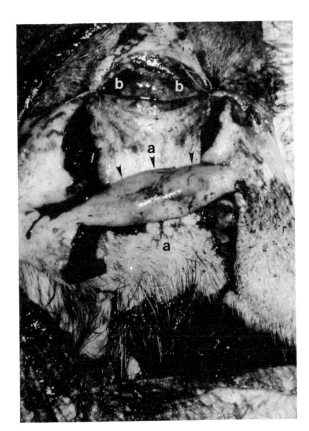

   e) Close the skin with 6-0 or 7-0 mersilene (Ethicon).
   f) Allow this to remain for 2 weeks, then perform reconstructive surgery.
    (1) Incise parallel to the lid margin, through the skin and muscle *to*—not through—the conjunctiva.
    (2) Undermine the conjunctiva to provide an apron longer than the skin and muscle.
    (3) Suture the conjunctiva to the skin edge, providing a mucosal surface on the edge.
    (4) Repair the ventral lid defect.
     i) Freshen the cut edge of the free lid.
     ii) Reappose the two margins.
     iii) Suture conjunctiva to conjunctiva with 7-0 chromic gut.
     iv) Close the skin with 6-0 or 7-0 mersilene (Ethicon).
   g) Remove the skin sutures in 10 to 14 days.
  2. Ventral lid defects—a simple V-plasty is effective (p. 84)
  3. Other procedures for agenesis reconstructive surgeries are listed in Suggested Readings.
 F. Prognosis—fair to excellent, depending on severity

II. Dermoids
 A. General
  1. Ectopic islands of skin on:
   a) Conjunctiva
   b) Cornea
   c) Can be associated with lid "colobomas" in dogs (above)
 B. Etiology—unknown
 C. Clinical signs
  1. Visible island of ectopic skin
  2. Blepharospasms
  3. Epiphora
  4. Possible ulcerative keratoconjunctivitis
 D. Diagnosis—by observation
 E. Treatment
  1. Surgical excision
  2. Subsequent repair of resulting defect
 F. Prognosis—excellent

III. Defects of the cilia or periocular hair
 A. Distichiasis (Fig. 4-7)
  1. General
   a) Common in dogs, particularly in some breeds
   b) Rare in cats
   c) Extra row of cilia, which arises from the tarsal (meibomian) gland ducts (Fig. 4-7, Table 4-1)
  2. Etiology—congenital, may be inherited

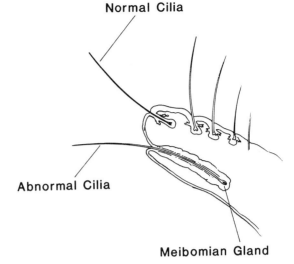

Normal Cilia

Abnormal Cilia

Meibomian Gland

Fig. 4-7. Schematic drawing demonstrating origin of abnormal cilia (distichiasis).

3. Clinical signs
   a) May observe hairs only without overt secondary ocular disease
      (1) Long, soft hairs may not cause problems
      (2) Short, stiff hairs cause corneal irritation
   b) Epiphora—most frequent sign
   c) Conjunctival erythema
   d) Blepharospasm
   e) Pannus
   f) Ulcerative keratitis
   g) The above lesions may be complicated, not caused, by distichiasis
4. Diagnosis
   a) Assess the lesions critically.
   b) Observe location of the hairs.
      (1) Place a white plastic spoon under the lid to demonstrate hairs.
      (2) Use indirect illumination and magnification.
5. Treatment
   a) To date, there is no panacea.
   b) Cryosurgery (Scagliotti's method) holds the most promise.
      (1) Anesthetize the animal.
      (2) Use a 2-mm cryoprobe with tip temperature at −80°C.
      (3) Hold the probe against the conjunctival surface adjacent to the tarsal gland containing the cilia.
      (4) Produce an ice ball and maintain it for 1 minute 15 seconds, then allow it to thaw slowly.
      (5) Move over several cilia and then repeat process.

TABLE 4-1. BREED PREDISPOSITION FOR OCULAR LESIONS

Atresia lacrimal puncta

  Bedlington terrier
  Cocker spaniel
    American
    English
  Poodle
    Miniature
    Toy
  Schnauzer, miniature
  Sealyham terrier
  Persian cats

Cataracts (see Table 12-1)

Chronic superficial keratitis (degenerative
    pannus)

  Dachshund, miniature, standard
  German shepherd
  Greyhound
  Poodle, miniature

Collie eye anomaly

  Collie
  German shepherd (?)
  Shetland sheepdog

Corneal dystrophy

  Epithelial or superficial stroma

    Airedale
    Afghan
    Akita
    Alaskan malamute
    Bichon Frise
    Boston terrier
    Cocker spaniel
    Collie
    Dachshund
    German shepherd
    Irish setter
    Poodle
      Miniature
      Toy
    Pug
    Schnauzer, miniature
    Shetland sheepdog
    Wirehaired fox terrier

Corneal dystrophy (*continued*)

  Endothelial

    Boston terrier
    Boxer
    Chihuahua
    Cocker spaniel
    Dachshund
    Poodle, miniature
    Wirehaired fox terrier

  Epithelial erosion–indolent ulcer (basement
    membrane dystrophy?)

    Boston terrier
    Boxer
    Dachshund
    Poodle, miniature
    Welsh corgi
    Wirehaired terrier

  Stromal dystrophy (deep)

    Siberian husky
    Manx cats

Distichiasis

  Bedlington terrier
  Boston terrier
  Boxer
  Cocker spaniel
    American
    English
  English bulldog
  English springer spaniel
  Great Dane
  Golden retriever
  Irish setter
  Labrador retriever
  Norwegian elkhound
  Old English sheepdog
  Pekingese
  Pomeranian
  Poodles
    Miniature
    Toy
  Pugs
  Shetland sheepdog
  Abyssinian cats

(*continued*)

TABLE 4-1. (*Continued*)

Ectropion

Basset hound
Beagle
Bloodhound
Clumber spaniel
Cocker spaniel
  American
  English
English bulldog
Newfoundland
Saint Bernard
Springer spaniel

Entropion

Boston terrier
Chesapeake Bay retriever
Chow chow
Cocker spaniel
  American
  English
Collie
Doberman pinscher
English bulldog
German shorthair pointer
Golden retriever
Gordon setter
Great Dane
Irish setter
Kerry blue terrier
Labrador retriever
Lhasa apso
Newfoundland
Pekingese
Poodle
  Miniature
  Toy
Pug
Rottweiler
Saint Bernard
Schnauzer, miniature
Shar-pei
Shih Tzu
Persian cats

Everted cartilage

Bull Mastiff
Chesapeake Bay retriever
Doberman pinscher
German shepherd
German shorthair pointer
Great Dane
Newfoundland
Saint Bernard
Weimaraner

Glaucoma

Australian shepherd (blue healer)
Afghan hound
Basset hound
Beagle
Cocker spaniel
  American
  English
Jack Russell terrier
Norwegian elkhound
Poodle
  Miniature
  Toy
Sealyham terrier
Smooth fox terrier
Tibetan terrier
Welsh corgi terrier
Wirehaired fox terrier

Hypertrophy of the nictitan gland (Cherry
  Eye)

Basset hound
Beagle
Boston terrier
Cocker spaniel
  American
  English

Hypoplasia optic nerve (hypoplasia ganglion
  cells)

Beagle
Dachshund
Poodle, miniature
Saint Bernard

Keratoconjunctivitis sicca

Chihuahua
Dachshund, miniature
English bulldog
Schnauzer, miniature
West Highland terrier

Lagophthalmos

Pekingese
Pug

Lens luxation or subluxation

Jack Russell terrier
Sealyham terrier
Smooth fox terrier
Tibetan terrier
Welsh corgi terrier
Wirehaired fox terrier

(*continued*)

TABLE 4-1 *(Continued)*

Microphthalmia

  Australian shepherd
  Collie
  Dalmation
  Great Dane
  Poodle
    Miniature
    Toy
  Schnauzer, miniature

Persistent hyperplastic primary vitreous

  Doberman pinscher
  Schnauzer, miniature

Persistent pupillary membranes

  Afghan hound
  Australian shepherd
  Basenji
  Basset hound
  Beagle
  Chow chow
  Cocker spaniel
    American
    English
  Collie
  Dachshund
  Doberman pinscher
  English bulldog
  English springer spaniel
  Great Pyrenees
  Irish setter
  Pembroke corgi
  Rottweiler
  Saluki
  Samoyed
  Schnauzer, miniature
  Scottish terrier
  Shetland sheepdog
  Siberian husky
  Tibetan terrier
  Welsh corgi

Retinal atrophy
  Central progressive retinal atrophy

    Briard
    Labrador retriever
    Shetland sheepdog

  Gyrate atrophy of retina and choroid

    Mixed breeds of cats

Hemeralopia

  Alaskan malamute
  Poodle, miniature
  White German shepherd (?)

Progressive cone-rod degeneration

  Standard poodle

Progressive retinal atrophy

  Akita
  Belgian shepherd
  Cardigan Welsh corgi
  Chesapeake Bay retriever
  Cocker spaniel
    American
    English
  Collie
  Golden retriever
  Irish setter
  Labrador retriever
  Norwegian elkhound (early and late
    onset)
  Poodle, miniature
  Samoyed
  Schnauzer, miniature
  Tibetan terrier
  Abyssinian cats (?)
  Mixed breeds cats (?)
  Persian cats (?)
  Siamese cats (?)

Retinal dysplasia

  Focal, multifocal

    Cocker spaniel
      American
      English
    English springer spaniel
    Labrador retriever

  Generalized

    Bedlington terrier
    Labrador retriever
    Sealyham terrier
    Yorkshire terrier

  Associated with multiple ocular anomalies

    Australian shepherd
    Great Dane
    Dalmatian
    Labrador retriever

(continued)

TABLE 4-1. (*Continued*)

Spontaneous retinal detachment	Tapetal hypoplasia
Dachshund, miniature Poodle, miniature	Beagle
Stationary nightblindness (?)	Trichiasis (deviation of the upper lateral cilia)
Briard Tibetan terrier	Chihuahua Kerry blue terrier Pekingese
Strabismus	Pomeranian Pug
Siamese cats	Toy fox terrier

(6) This may be done in several areas and repeated in 2 or 3 weeks when entire lid is involved.

(7) After operation:

   i) The lids become erythematous and edematous.

   ii) Warm compresses should be applied two or three times per day.

   iii) Systemic antibiotics should be given for 1 week.

   iv) Systemic prednisone 0.5 mg/kg bid for 2 days, then 0.25 mg/kg bid for the remainder of 1 week

   v) Poliosis will result in a few weeks.

  6. Prognosis

    a) Procedure is too new to be evaluated critically, but it shows great promise (see Suggested Readings).

    b) A guarded prognosis must still be given.

B. Ectopic cilia

  1. General

    a) Often missed cause of corneal ulceration

    b) Can originate from upper or lower lids (Fig. 4-8)

  2. Etiology—basically unknown

    a) Acquired—my belief

    b) Inherited—no evidence

  3. Clinical signs

    a) Recurring superficial, well-circumscribed ulcerative keratitis

      (1) Circular

      (2) Linear

    b) Pain—usually severe

      (1) Epiphora

      (2) Blepharospasms

      (3) Enophthalmos

      (4) Prolapse of the third eyelid

      (5) Head jerk at the height of the blink

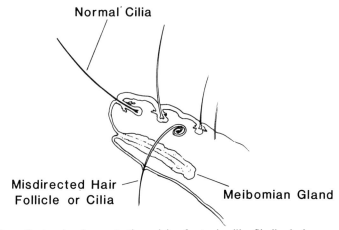

Fig. 4-8. Schematic drawing demonstrating origin of ectopic cilia. Similar lesions can result from aberrant growth and misdirection of lid hair, also.

   c) Hair on the palpebral surface—requires magnification (Fig. 4-9)
    (1) Single stiff, bristly hair
    (2) Reddish, blister-like swelling with many shafts of hair
  4. Diagnosis
   a) Clinical signs
   b) Observing hair(s)
  5. Treatment
   a) Simple epilation is my preference.
   b) All of the hairs must be removed.
   c) Some advocate surgical excision.
   d) Secondary ulcerative keratitis is treated as an uncomplicated ulcer (see p. 159—Cornea).
  6. Prognosis—excellent when hairs are removed permanently
 C. Trichiasis—aberrant lashes directed toward the cornea (see Table 4-1)
  1. General
   a) Best exemplified by deviation of the lateral cilia observed in Chihuahuas, toy fox terriers, Kerry blue terriers, Pekingeses, Pomeranians, and pugs (Fig. 4-10)
   b) Not entropion, but deviated cilia only
   c) In veterinary medicine, all periocular hair is placed in this category (see Redundant nasal folds, Caruncular trichiasis)
  2. Etiology—most of the defects are inherited or presumed inherited
  3. Clinical signs
   a) Upper lateral cilia are misdirected toward the cornea.
   b) Most often bilateral

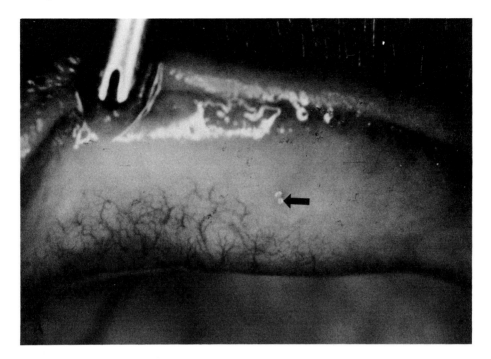

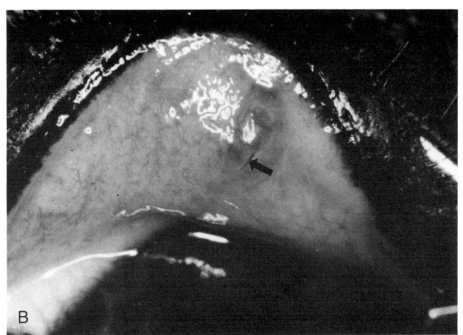

Fig. 4-9. Ectopic cilia from upper palpebral conjunctival surface (arrow). (A) Young Doberman female with bilateral ectopic cilia. (B) Four-year old Shih-Tzu male with ectopic cilia of upper the lid (arrow). Notice the swollen appearance.

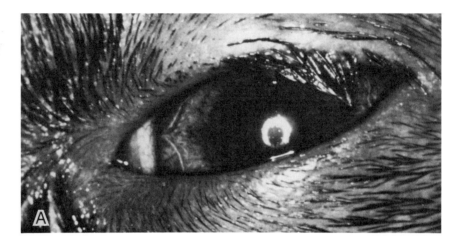

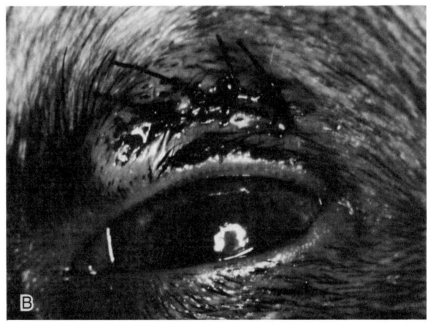

Fig. 4-10. Pomeranian puppy demonstrating deviated lateral cilia. (A) Before operation. (B) After operation.

    c) Results in corneal disease due to mechanical irritation.
       (1) Blepharospasm
       (2) Epiphora
       (3) Conjunctival erythema
       (4) Periocular soiling
       (5) Ulcerative keratitis

         4. Diagnosis—by observation
         5. Treatment—modified Hotz–Celsus procedure (p. 82) (Fig. 4-10)
         6. Prognosis—excellent
   D. Redundant nasal folds—rarely a cause of corneal irritation
         1. Etiology—breed predispostion
         2. Clinical signs
           a) Similar to any chronic irritation
           b) Observe nasal fold hair contacting cornea
           c) Pannus
           d) Ulcerative keratitis
         3. Diagnosis—by observation
         4. Treatment—surgical excision of nasal fold (see Suggested Readings)
         5. Prognosis—generally good
   E. Caruncular trichiasis
         1. General
           a) Often missed by the practitioner
           b) Frequently occurs in poodles, Pekingese, Shih-Tzus, and pugs
         2. Clinical signs
           a) Long, resilient hairs emanating from the caruncle
           b) Acts as a wick, causing the weepy dog syndrome
           c) Causes pannus (pigmentary keratitis)
           d) Ulcerative keratitis—rare
           e) Rarely causes pain
         3. Diagnosis—by observation
         4. Treatment
           a) Surgical excision of the caruncle
           b) Cryotherapy—used by several veterinary ophthalmologists to destroy the hair follicles
             (1) Anesthetize the animal.
             (2) Place the cryoprobe on the caruncle, forming an ice ball; maintain for 2 minutes.
             (3) Thaw slowly.
             (4) Repeat until the entire caruncle has been frozen, which destroys the germinal center of hair.
             (5) Swelling occurs 12 to 24 hours after therapy.
             (6) Conjunctival erythema and chemosis occur after therapy.
             (7) Poliosis is an expected sequella.
IV. Entropion—common in dogs, less common in cats (see Table 4-1)
   A. Three forms
         1. Congenital—inherited
           a) Entropion—Predisposing conditions
             (1) Large orbit
                i) Results in deeply set eye.
                ii) Does not provide adequate lid support.

  iii) Space between orbital rim and the eye is greater than normal.
  iv) Lid "droops" over lower orbital rim, resulting in inversion.
   v) Predisposed breeds include the collie, Doberman pinscher, golden retriever, Great Dane, Irish setter, rottweiler, and weimaraner.
(2) Defect in muscular development
  i) Not well documented
  ii) Retractor anguli oculi muscle is said to be poorly developed.
  iii) Results in a rounded lateral canthus
  iv) Predisposed breeds include the Chesapeake Bay retriever, chow chow, and Samoyed.
(3) Primary lid deformity
  i) Poorly understood
  ii) Requires basic research to define more clearly
  iii) Predisposed breeds include the Airedale, basset hound, bloodhound, bullmastiff, cocker spaniel, curly-coated Retriever, English bulldog, English setter, German short-haired pointer, Kerry blue terrier, Labrador retriever, mastiff, Newfoundland, Old English sheepdog, pointer, Pyrenean mountain dog, Saint Bernard, schipperke, Shar-pei, and springer spaniel
  iv) Reported in Persian cats
b) Medial entropion
(1) In addition to the general signs of entropion there is (pigment) infiltration of the medial cornea
(2) Caruncular hairs are common in this group.
(3) Predisposed breeds include the Boston terrier, Lhasa apso, Pekingese, miniature pinscher, miniature and toy poodle, pug, and Shih-Tzu
2. Acquired nonspastic
a) Cause—not inherited
(1) Surgery
(2) Trauma resulting in scars
(3) Chronic inflammatory cicatricial entropion
b) Usually unilateral
c) Often historical evidence related to lesion
3. Acquired spastic
a) Most common type observed in cats
b) Etiologies—usually associated with painful corneal and/or conjunctival disease
c) Usually unilateral
B. Clinical signs (see Fig. A-1)

      1. Severity is variable
      2. Rolling in of the lid margin(s) with lid hairs exhibiting a white or grayish coating
      3. Epiphora
      4. Chemosis
      5. Conjunctival erythema
      6. Conjunctivitis
      7. Blepharospasm
      8. Pain
      9. Corneal ulceration and its sequellae
    10. Photophobia
C. Diagnosis
      1. By observation
      2. Critical evaluation of lesions to categorize entropion
D. Treatment
      1. Each patient must be evaluated and treated individually.
      2. Evaluation
         a) Determine the cause and classification.
         b) Critically evaluate each eye while the patient is awake.
         c) Decide which surgical procedure is most acceptable for that patient.
      3. Methods for repair
         a) Temporary vertical mattress sutures
            (1) May be successful in treating spastic entropion or in very young animals (e.g., Shar-peis)
            (2) Use two or three 4-0 mersilene (Ethicon) sutures to evert the involved lid.
            (3) Place sutures close to the lid margin into tarsal plate and perpendicular to free lid margin.
            (4) Take second bite away from the lid into the skin.
            (5) Apply adequate tension to evert the lid margin.
            (6) Leave for 2 to 4 weeks.
         b) Correcting for a large orbital rim—lateral canthoplasty
            (1) Perform a lateral tarsectomy.
            (2) Remove an adequate amount of tarsal plate to shorten the lid and tighten the palpebral margin.
            (3) Cut free lid margin at a 45° angle, directed toward the lateral canthus.
            (4) Tailor the amount to the patient.
            (5) Continue the incision from the upper to the lower lid.
            (6) Close the conjunctiva with a running mattress suture (see V-plasty).
            (7) Reform the lateral canthus meticulously.
                i) Place intrastromal mattress sutures to reform the lateral canthus—use 5-0 or 6-0 mersilene (Ethicon).

      ii) Close the remaining defect with simple interrupted sutures.
- (8) Remove the sutures in 7 to 10 days.
- (9) This method is not acceptable for an exophthalmic eye predisposed to lagophthalmos.
- c) Correcting a defect in muscular development
  - (1) Lateral canthoplasty
  - (2) See Suggested Readings
- d) Correcting for primary lid deformity
  - (1) Modified Hotz–Celsus technique
    - i) Excise an elliptical piece of skin adjacent to the entropic lid.
    - ii) Make an incision with a #15 Bard Parker blade.
    - iii) Make the first incision as close as possible to the tarsal plate without invading it.
    - iv) Make the second incision a gentle elipse, the widest part of which is determined before anesthesia is induced.
    - v) To determine the amount to be removed:
      - (A) Place the thumb on the lid skin and pull down until the free lid margin is observed.
      - (B) The distance moved is the amount of tissue to remove at the widest part of the eliptical piece of skin.
      - (C) Extend the length 1 mm on either side of the deviatcd lid margin.
    - vi) Closure
      - (A) Close with simple interrupted 5-0 or 6-0 mersilene (Ethicon) sutures.
      - (B) Place the sutures in an arrow pattern (Fig. 4-11).
      - (C) Direct the arrow toward the free lid margin.
      - (D) The pattern accentuates eversion.
      - (E) Remove the sutures in 7 to 10 days.
  - (2) Tarsal pedicles
    - i) Make the skin incision parallel to the free lid margin, just below the tarsus adjacent to the inverted lid.
    - ii) Elevate the incision at the free lid margin.
    - iii) Identify the tarsus and form a tarsal pedicle attached close to the free lid margin.
    - iv) Undermine the opposite margin, forming a pocket; place the tarsal pedicle into the pocket.
    - v) Grasp the pedicle at its free border and transfix the base with 5-0 or 4-0 double-armed mersilene (Ethicon). Continue with a cruciate pattern, exiting at the free margin.

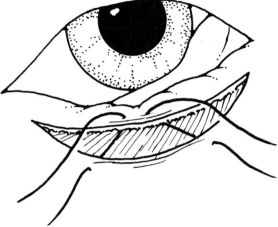

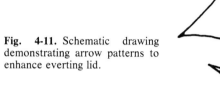

Fig. 4-11. Schematic drawing demonstrating arrow patterns to enhance everting lid.

      vi) Place sutures into the fashioned pocket, exiting the skin, and tie externally over a rubber stint

      vii) Excise the skin that overlaps at the primary incision, and close the resulting defect as in the Hotz–Celsus technique.

      viii) The number of pedicles necessary to correct the problem varies depending on the severity of the lid defect(s).

V. Ectropion forms (see Table 4-1)
- A. Physiologic
  1. Natural breed characteristic in basset hounds, bloodhounds, clumber spaniels, cocker spaniels, English bulldogs, and Saint Bernards
  2. No overt associated corneal or conjunctival disease
- B. Pathologic
  1. Congenital
     - a) Occurs in the same breeds as the physiologic form, but ocular disease is manifest
     - b) Etiology—inherited
     - c) Clinical signs
       - (1) Everted lids
       - (2) Conjunctivitis
       - (3) Epiphora
       - (4) Keratitis—usually due to exposure
       - (5) Purulent exudate
  2. Acquired
     - (1) Three forms
       - i) Intermittent
         - (A) Cause—myasthenia of the facial and ocular muscles in hunting dogs

  (*B*) Clinical signs
   (*1*) Same as for congenital form, but not as severe
   (*2*) Intermittent—appearing late in the day
 ii) Senile
  (*A*) Etiology—age in predisposed breeds (see p. 83—
   Physiologic ectropion)
   (*1*) Atrophy of lid muscles
   (*2*) Myasthenia
  (*B*) Clinical signs
   (*1*) Variable
   (*2*) Depend on the degree of ectropion
 iii) Cicatricial ectropion
  (*A*) Etiology
   (*1*) Sequela to overcorrection of entropion
   (*2*) Trauma resulting in adherent scars everting lids
  (*B*) Clinical signs
   (*1*) Similar to those described under congenital pathologic clinical signs
   (*2*) Identification of scars
   (*3*) Usually unilateral
(2) Treatment
 i) Establish classification
 ii) Shorten the lid for congenital eversion
  (*A*) V-plasty
   (*1*) Remove a V-shaped portion of the affected lid large enough to shorten the lid adequately.
   (*2*) Excise laterally, staying in tarsal plate.
   (*3*) Perform closure in two layers.
   (*4*) Close the conjunctiva with a continuous running mattress of 6-0 or 7-0 chromic gut—start at the apex moving toward the free margin.
   (*5*) Close the free lid margin meticulously.
    (*a*) Place intratarsal mattress suture using 5-0 or 6-0 mersilene (Ethicon).
    (*b*) Close the remaining wound routinely, with simple interrupted sutures.
   (*6*) Remove sutures in 7 to 10 days.
  (*B*) Lateral blepharoplasty (see Suggested Readings)
   (*1*) Shortens the lid without producing a scar in the free lid margin
   (*2*) Digital pressure laterally determines the amount necessary to shorten the lid margin
   (*3*) Prepare the animal for surgery.

(4) Make an incision at the lateral canthus, continuing the arc of the lower lid 2 mm longer than the predetermined amount to shorten the lid.

(5) Make a second incision continuing the arc of the upper lid for the lower lid.

(6) Connect the two arms forming an arching triangle. Remove this skin.

(7) Perform a tarsectomy to the lateral canthus, including all of the lateral canthus.

(8) Reform the lateral canthus with an intrastromal suture pattern.

(9) Move the triangle dorsolaterally and close with simple interrupted sutures.

iii) Relieve the scar for cicatricial ectropion with a V-Y plasty

(A) Prepare the animal routinely.

(B) Identify the extent of the scar.

(C) Make a V incision encompassing the scar.

(D) Undermine the skin flap toward the free lid margin, relieving scar adhesions.

(E) Close the resulting lesion with simple interrupted 5-0 or 6-0 mersilene (Ethicon) suture in the form of a Y.

(F) This allows the free lid margin to move toward the eye.

INFLAMMATORY DISEASES (BLEPHARITIS) (see Fig. A-1)

I. Common in all animals

II. Etiologies
  A. Bacteria
  B. Fungi
  C. Parasites
  D. Allergies
  E. Photosensitivities
  F. Endocrinopathies
  G. Immune-mediated diseases

III. Clinical signs
  A. May be generalized or focal, affecting one or both lids of either eye
  B. Blepharospasm
  C. Blepharoedema
  D. Hyperemia
  E. Excoriation

    F. Poliosis
    G. Pruritis, self-mutilation
    H. Exudates
    I. Epiphora
    J. Bleeding
    K. Squamous detritus
    L. Thickened keratosis
    M. Focal swellings
    N. Alopecia
IV. Diagnosis
    A. Clinical signs
    B. Careful examination
    C. Exfoliative cytology or impression smear
    D. Culture
    E. Biopsies
 V. Specific diseases
    A. Hordeolum (stye)
       1. Internal—inflammation of the meibomian glands (meibomianitis)
       2. External—inflammation of the lash follicle or gland of Zeis
       3. Most often a bacterial infection—*Staphylococcus aureus* is most common
       4. Clinical signs
         a) Acute
         b) Painful
         c) Red swellings at the free lid margin
         d) Puppies
           (1) Multiple swellings throughout all lids
           (2) May be a modification of "puppy strangles"
       5. Treatment
         a) Drainage
           (1) Anesthetize the animal.
           (2) Puncture the swelling with a 25- to 20-gauge needle.
           (3) Gently express the abcess.
           (4) Results in marked swelling—client should be forewarned.
         b) Hot compresses—15 minutes per time bid or tid
         c) Systemic antibiotics—ampicillin 20 mg/kg tid
         d) Low doses of steroids—0.25d to 0.50 mg/kg divided bid
       6. Prognosis—generally excellent
    B. Chalazion—chronic inflammation and distention of a meibomian gland
       1. General
         a) Not an infection, a distention of the gland
         b) Most often observed in older dogs and, less frequently, in cats
         c) Often confused with lid neoplasms
       2. Clinical signs
         a) Nonpainful swellings on palpebral conjunctiva

b) Secondary conjunctival disease may be presenting sign
3. Diagnosis
   a) Clinical signs
   b) By observation
4. Treatment
   a) Anesthetize the animal.
   b) Fix the involved gland in a chalazion forceps.
   c) Evert the lid and incise it over the swelling.
     (1) Use a #11 Bard Parker blade.
     (2) Make the incision perpendicular to free lid margin.
     (3) Currettage (chalazion curette)
   d) Give systemic antibiotics for 5 to 7 days.
   e) Warm compresses may be indicated.
4. Prognosis—good to excellent
C. Bacterial blepharitis
1. Etiology—many bacteria, with *Staphylococcus* most common
2. Clinical signs
   a) Acute
     (1) Bilateral or unilateral
     (2) Blepharospasm
     (3) Hyperemia
     (4) Variable amounts of exudate
     (5) Encrustations, excoriation
   b) Chronic
     (1) Ulceration
     (2) Alopecia
     (3) Medial canthal erosion (usually a *Staphylococcus* blepharitis)
     (4) I believe chronic staphylococcal infections:
       i) Elaborate necrotizing toxins.
       ii) Sensitize the skin to the toxins or organisms that produce necrosis.
3. Diagnosis
   a) Clinical signs
   b) Culture
   c) Biopsy
4. Treatment
   a) Appropriate systemic antibiotic(s)
   b) For medial canthal erosion, systemic steroids 0.5 mg/kg divided bid
   c) Some advocate autogenous vaccines—my experience indicates little efficacy with this method
   d) Gentle cleansing and warm compresses
   e) Eliminate seborrhea or other systemic endocrinopathies affecting the skin

D. Parasitic blepharitis
 1. Etiologies
   a) *Notedres cati* (cats)
   b) *Sarcoptes* (dogs)
   c) Demodecticosis—more common in dogs than in cats
 2. Clinical signs
   a) Unilateral or bilateral
   b) Hyperemia
   c) Scaliness
   d) Alopecia
   e) Pruritis—particularly *Sarcoptes*
 3. Diagnosis
   a) Clinical signs
   b) Scrapings are diagnostic
 4. Treatment
   a) Similar to generalized parasitic dermatitis
   b) Local bid application of one of the following:
     (1) Rotenone
     (2) Sulfur
     (3) Isoflurophate ophthalmic ointments
   c) Protective collars are prudent
 5. Prognosis—poor to good
E. Dermatomycotic blepharitis
 1. Etiologies:
   a) *Microsporum canis*
   b) *Trichophyton mentagraphytes*
   c) Rarely do other mycoses affect the lids of dogs and cats
 2. Clinical signs
   a) Alopecia
   b) Hyperemia
   c) Blepharedema
   d) Scaliness
 3. Diagnosis
   a) Clinical signs
   b) Direct microscopic examination from skin scrapings treated
      with potassium hydroxide
   c) Wood's light examination—helpful for *Microsporum* spp
 4. Treatment—50 mg/kg/day griseofulvin PO
 5. Prognosis—good to excellent
F. Allergic blepharitis—more research is needed to better define this
   category
 1. Etiologies—acute reactions from:
   a) Vaccination
   b) Drugs—angioneurotic edema
   c) Insect bites

        d) Sunlight exposure
    2. See Suggested Readings
  G. Canine allergic inhalant dermatitis (CAID, Atopy)
    1. Etiology—Dogs with CAID form IgE antibodies against many antigens that are innocuous to nonallergic dogs
    2. Clinical signs
      a) Both sexes may be affected.
      b) Age—lesions are manifest most frequently in animals 12 to 36 months old but can occur at any age
      c) Erythema
      d) Swelling
      e) Encrustations
      f) Scaling
      g) Excoriation
      h) Increased pigmentation
      i) Lichenification
      j) Severe pruritis
    3. Diagnosis
      a) History and examination—very important
      b) Identify allergen(s)—skin testing
      c) Biopsies
    4. Treatment
      a) Must obtain specific diagnosis before treating
      b) Corticosteroids—not a panacea
      c) Immunotherapy (hyposensitization) (see Suggested Readings for techniques)
    5. Prognosis—guarded
  H. Autoimmune complex—pemphigus group (vulgaris in dogs and cats; foliaceus, erythematosus, and vegetatus in dogs only)
    1. Most common diseases—ocular lesions are rarely seen alone
      a) Vulgaris
        (1) Severe involvement at mucocutaneous junction
        (2) Acute intraepidermal bulla
        (3) Clinical febrile systemic illness
        (4) Secondary bacterial infections common
      b) Foliaceus
        (1) Superficial bulla
        (2) Scaling
        (3) Alopecia
        (4) Encrustation
        (5) Pruritis
    2. Most often observed in animals 1 year of age or older
    3. Hyperkeratosis of the pads may be a helpful diagnostic sign
    4. Diagnosis
      a) Clinical signs

b) Biopsies
(1) Microscopic examination
i) Vulgaris—suprabasilar cleft formation with acantholysis
ii) Foliaceus—subcorneal bulla with acantholysis
(2) Immunofluorescence—epidermal intercellular deposits of IgG and C3 seen on direct immunofluorescence
5. Treatment
a) Immunosuppressive corticosteroid—dose is 1 to 2 mg/kg prednisilone divided bid
b) Systemic antibiotics
c) Potential immunosuppressive agents
(1) Cyclophosphamide 2 mg/kg once daily 4 days per week
(2) Azathioprine 2 mg/kg daily
(3) CBC and urinalysis should be monitored for bone marrow suppression and hemorrhagic cystitis
6. Prognosis—guarded
I. Bullous pemphigoid—acute (most severe) or chronic
1. Clinical signs
a) Similar to pemphigus vulgaris, without rupture of the bulla
b) Observed at mucotaneous junctions
c) Secondary bacterial infection is common
2. Diagnosis—requires examination of biopsy specimen
a) Histopathologic examination identifies inflammatory cell colonization of subepidermal clefts.
b) Direct immunofluorescence identifies immunoglobulin deposits around the basement membrane; these may be absent in the chronic form.
3. Treatment
a) Same as for the pemphigus group, but less aggressive
b) Localized lesions are often responsive to local steroid/antibiotic therapy
4. Prognosis—good to fair
J. Lupus erythematosus
1. Discoid (DLE)
a) Has been described in dogs but not unanimously accepted
b) Benign and usually limited to the skin
2. Systemic (SLE)
a) 30% to 50% of SLE patients have skin lesions
b) Lid lesions—"batwing" or "butterfly" appearance around eyes and bridge of nose
c) Erythema
d) Alopecia
e) Scaling
f) Crusting
g) Atrophy

       h) Scarring
       i) Vesicles and bullae may erode, causing ulceration
       j) Pruritis
   3. Diagnosis
       a) Clinical signs and history
       b) LE tests are helpful but of limited value, especially for DLE.
       c) ANA may be helpful in SLE but usually is negative in DLE.
       d) Histopathologic evaluations are the most reliable diagnostic aids.
   4. Treatment
       a) Immunosuppressive corticosteroid—dose is 1 to 2 mg/kg prednisilone divided bid
       b) Antimalarial drugs have been advocated for DLE—hydroxychloroquine sulfate 0.5 mg/kg/day until improvement is observed

K. Iatrogenic allergic blepharitis (more accurately, blepharoconjunctivitis)—rare in dogs and cats
   1. Etiology—usually associated with topical therapy
   2. Clinical signs (Fig. 4-12)
       a) Severe erythema
       b) Excoriation
       c) Alopecia
       d) Erosive conjunctivitis
       e) Sometimes keratitis
       f) Rhinitis
       g) Glossitis
       h) Errosion of the lips
       i) History of treating eye topically
   3. Diagnosis
       a) Clinical signs
       b) History—exacerbation with treatment
       c) Biopsies—predominant cell types are lymphocytes, plasma cells, and eosinophils
   4. Treatment
       a) Once diagnosis is made, allergen is eliminated
       b) No topical therapy is indicated
   5. Prognosis—excellent

LAGOPHTHALMOS

I. Etiologies
  A. Exophthalmos
    1. Occurs as a result of constant pressure on the lids by the prominent eye

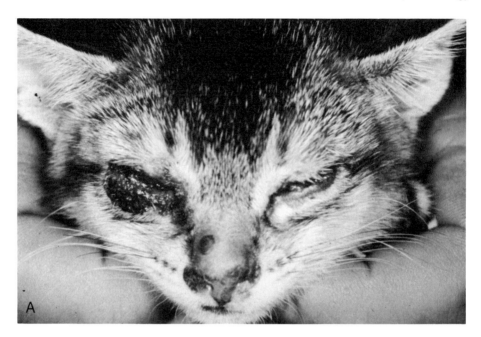

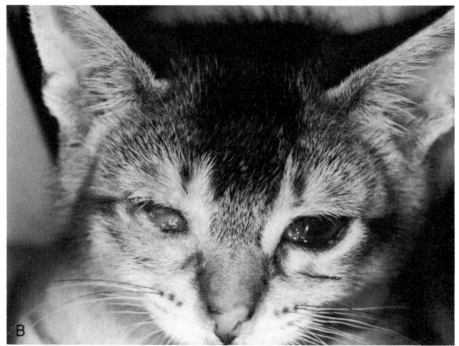

Fig. 4-12. Abyssinian kitten with drug-induced keratoconjunctivitis. (A) Before terminating a rigorous topical medical regimen. Bacterial and viral cultures were negative; cytologic study demonstrated plasma cells, eosinophils, and lymphocytes as the predominant cell population. (B) Ten days after all topical medication was discontinued.

      2. Results in enlargement of the palpebral fissure and subsequent inability to close the eye
      3. Predisposed breeds include pugs, Pekingese, and Shi-Tzu
      4. Most frequently observed in older dogs
   B. Facial nerve palsy
      1. Trauma
      2. Otitis media
      3. Chronic hypothyroidism
      4. Pituitary neoplasia
II. Clinical signs
   A. Lagophthalmos
      1. Prominent eye
      2. Fifth nerve stimulation results in a weak or partial blink
      3. The axial or periaxial cornea is usually eroded.
         a) Keratomalacia
         b) Descemetocele
         c) Neovasculalrization
         d) Cellular infiltration
         e) May be dry (lusterless)
         f) Pannus
         g) Anterior uveitis
           (1) Frequently severe
           (2) Hypopyon
           (3) Hypotony
           (4) Flare
           (5) Miosis
           (6) Syenchiae
           (7) Blindness
   B. Facial nerve palsy
      1. Asymmetry of:
         a) Ears—auricular palpebral branch
         b) Eyelids—auricular palpebral branch
         c) Lips—buccal branch
         d) Nose (not very significant in dog and cat)
      2. Lagophthalmos
      3. Pannus
      4. Severe purulent keratoconjunctivitis
      5. Ulcerative keratitis
      6. Dry eye
III. Diagnosis
   A. Lagophthalmos
      1. Clinical signs
      2. Breed predisposition
   B. Facial nerve palsy
      1. Clinical signs

        2. Neurologic examination

        3. Ear examination

IV. Treatment

    A. Lagophthalmos—surgery

        1. Medial permanent tarsorrhaphy

        2. Lateral permanent tarsorrhaphy

        3. Both

    B. Facial nerve palsy

        1. According to some authors, a steroid-responsive transient hemoparesis occurs

        2. Must identify cause and treat specifically

        3. Permanent lateral tarsorrhaphy

        4. Tear supplementation

        5. Antibiotic topically

TRAUMA

  I. Common in dogs and cats (Fig. 4-13)

 II. Etiologies

    A. Bite wounds

    B. Cuts and abrasions

III. Clinical signs

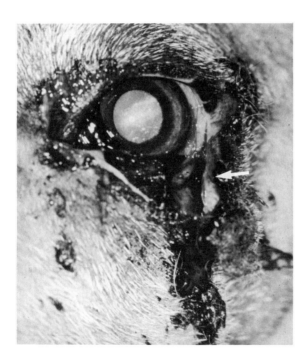

Fig. 4-13. Lower lid laceration in a dog. Arrow identifies ventral lid lesion in the left eye.

    A. Usually presents as an acute problem
    B. The torn lid is clinically demonstrable.
    C. The affected lid is swollen and bruised.
    D. Conjunctivitis and chemosis
    E. Bloody discharge
    F. May have corneal involvement
 IV. Diagnosis—by observation
  V. Treatment
    A. Evaluate the patient for shock and treat appropriately.
    B. Induce general anesthesia.
    C. Irrigate with warm physiologic saline—may use dental pic.
    D. Shave perilesional hair
    E. Debride minimally.
    F. Reconstruct lid.
      1. Must be done in tissue plains
      2. Close conjunctiva from apex to free border with continuous (7-0 chromic gut) mattress suture in fibrous tissue layer of conjunctiva.
      3. Close lid skin starting at free lid margin and progressing toward apex of tear.
        a) Make a small intratarsal mattress suture with 5-0 or 6-0 non-absorbable suture.
        b) Close the remaining wound with simple, interrupted sutures.
    G. Remove sutures in 7 to 10 days.
 VI. Prognosis
    A. Acute injury—excellent
    B. Varies depending on extent of trauma and duration of injury

NEOPLASMS

   I. In general, neoplasms are more common in older dogs than in cats. Eyelid neoplasms in cats are usually more destructive than in dogs.
  II. Dogs
    A. Sebaceous adenoma
    B. Sebaceous adenocarcinoma
    C. Squamous papilloma
    D. Melanoma
      1. Benign
      2. Malignant
    E. Fibrous histiocytoma
    F. Basal cell carcinoma
    G. Mastocytoma
    H. Squamous cell carcinoma
    I. Fibroma
    J. Others

III. Cats
    A. Squamous cell carcinoma (especially white cats)
    B. Sebaceous adenoma and adenocarcinoma
    C. Basal cell carcinoma
    D. Fibroma
    E. Fibrosarcoma
    F. Neurofibroma
    G. Neurofibrosarcoma
    H. Mast cell tumor
    I. Others
IV. Clinical signs
    A. Signs depend on size and biologic activity of neoplasm
    B. Most frequently observed sign is presence of an enlarging mass with or without excoriation
V. Diagnosis
    A. Clinical signs
    B. Biopsy
VI. Treatment
    A. Surgical excision
      1. Lid masses up to one-third the length of the lid may be excised.
        a) Major blepharoplastic reconstruction is not required.
        b) Simple V-plasty is effective.
      2. Technique
        a) Anesthetize the patient and prepare routinely for surgery.
        b) Excise the mass, including a small margin of normal tissue on both sides of mass.
        c) Extend the incision adequately to eliminate "bunching" of tissue distal to the free lid margin.
        d) Close conjunctiva and free lid margins (see p. 84—V-plasty).
        e) Submit the specimen for histologic diagnosis of the margin.
        f) Remove sutures in 7 to 10 days.
    B. Alternative methods
      1. Blepharoplastic procedures
      2. Radiation therapy
      3. Immunotherapy
      4. Cryosurgery
      5. High-frequency radio diatherapy

SUGGESTED READINGS

Anderson WN: Canine Allergic Inhalant Dermatitis. Ralston Purina Company, Checkerboard Square, St. Louis, 1982

Severin GA: Veterinary Ophthalmology Notes. 2nd. Ed. College of Veterinary Medicine, Colorado State University, Fort Collins, CO, 1976

Slatter DH: Fundamentals of Veterinary Ophthalmology. WB Saunders, Philadelphia, 1981

Theilen GH, Madewell BR: Veterinary Cancer Medicine. Lea and Febiger, Philadelphia, 1979

Wheeler CA, Severin GA: Cryosurgical epilation for the treatment of distichiasis in the dog and cat. JAAHA 20:877, 1984

Wyman M: Lateral canthoplasty. JAAHA 7:196, 1971

Wyman M: Ophthalmic surgery for the practitioner. p. 311. In Veterinary Clinics of North America. Small animal practice. Vol. 9:2, WB Saunders, Philadelphia, 1979

5

The Conjunctiva

ANATOMY AND PHYSIOLOGY

The conjunctiva lines the inner surface of the lids, both surfaces of the third eyelid, and the anterior surface of the globe, excluding the cornea. The portion covering the globe, the bulbar conjunctiva, is loosely attached, and that covering the lids, the palpebral conjunctiva, is firmly attached to the tarsus and less mobile than the bulbar conjunctiva. The junction of the two is called the fornix. The fold produces a sac, called the conjunctival sac, upper and lower. The third eyelid produces two sacs, an inner or bulbar sac and an outer or palpebral sac.

Histologically, the conjunctiva is composed of two layers, the epithelium, which is a nonkeratinized squamous epithelium containing goblet cells, and the substantia propria. The substantia propria is further divided into the superficial adenoid layer and the fibrous connective tissue layer. The adenoid layer is a fine fibrous network containing many lymphocytes, a few mast cells, and histiocytes. Some of the lymphocytes produce IgA, which obtains a secretory piece when it crosses the conjunctival epithelium. This antibody participates in mucosal resistance to infection in the normal animal.

The substantia propria is firmly attached to the tarsus and loosely attached to the globe, except at the limbal region. Here, the conjunctiva, Tenon's capsule, and the sclera are firmly attached to each other for a distance of 2 to 3 mm from the limbus. This must be taken into consideration when mobilizing the conjunctiva for a flap, because the incorporation of Tenon's capsule dooms the procedure to failure. The loosely attached conjunctiva overlying the globe accommodates ocular mobility. Both the superficial and the deep portions of the substantia propria contain blood vessels and lymphatics.

The palpebral conjunctival blood supply originates from the peripheral and marginal arcades of the lids, which arise from the nasal and lacrimal arteries of the lid. The bulbar conjunctiva is supplied by the anterior ciliary arteries. The superficial vessels become the limbal arcades and result in "budding" in response to corneal disease. Deep stromal corneal disease or anterior uveitis predisposes to deep corneal vascularization. These vessels are usually straight and darker-colored, in contrast to the branching, lighter-colored superficial vessels. The palpebral conjunctiva appears redder than the bulbar conjunctiva, because the palpebral conjunctival vessels enter perpendicular to the surface and branch in the superficial portion of the conjunctiva. This should be kept in mind when evaluating hyperemia, or "red eyes," since the palpebral surfaces, when everted, are normally red.

CONGENITAL DISEASES

Few congenital diseases involve only the conjunctiva; those that are associated with the lids or cornea are discussed in Chapter 4 and Chapter 8.

I. Dermoid
  A. Clinical signs
    1. Ectopic islands of skin, which may contain hair and other adnexal features
    2. Can be found anywhere on the conjunctiva and often encroach on the cornea (Fig. 5-1)
    3. Hair usually visible
    4. Epiphora
    5. Conjunctival irritation
    6. Keratitis
    7. Blepharospasm (variable and dependent on secondary lesions)
    8. Observed very shortly after eyes are opened
  B. Diagnosis
    1. Clinical signs
    2. Observation of the lesions
  C. Treatment—surgical excision and closure
    1. If the lesion is in the medial canthal area, the surgeon must avoid the lacrimal drainage apparatus.
    2. The lesions are most often superficial and uncomplicated.
  D. Prognosis—excellent

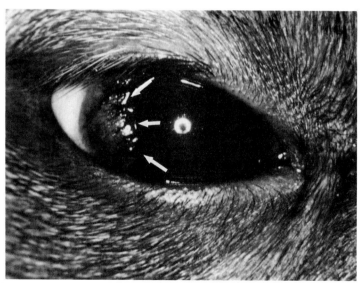

Fig. 5-1. Pomeranian puppy with a limbal dermoid (arrows), removed by superficial keratectomy and conjunctivectomy.

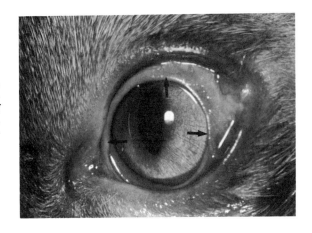

Fig. 5-2. Congenital symblepharon in an 8-month-old male Siamese cat. There was no history of previous inflammatory disease. Arrows indicate conjunctival margin encroaching on the cornea.

II. Congenital symblepharon—rare—I have observed it only in Siamese cats
   A. Clinical signs
      1. The eye appears smaller than normal because of the conjunctival fold.
      2. The bulbar conjunctiva has a fold that encircles the limbus and overlaps the cornea (Fig. 5-2)
      3. Variable epiphora
      4. Conjunctival hyperemia
   B. Diagnosis
      1. Clinical signs
      2. Identification of folds
   C. Treatment
      1. Make an incision at the lateral aspect of the defect.
      2. Retract the conjunctiva.
      3. Place 7-0 chromic gut sutures subconjunctivally, laterally to medially.
      4. The resulting lesion can be treated with topical antibiotics for 5 to 7 days.
   D. Prognosis
      1. Excellent
      2. May be inherited (speculative)
      3. The owner should be advised against breeding the animal(s).
III. Agenesis—occurs in conjunction with an absence of the lid (see p. 67).

INFLAMMATORY LESIONS

I. Bacterial conjunctivitis (see Fig. A-1)
   A. Dogs
      1. Etiologies

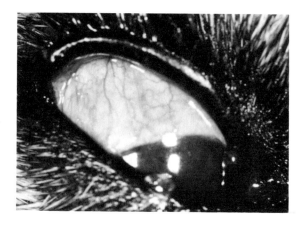

Fig. 5-3. Acute conjunctivitis in a 2-year-old female terrier cross. The lesion was unilateral, and the visible conjunctiva was moderately chemotic, red, and congested.

    a) *Staphylococcus aureus*
    b) *Streptococcus* spp
    c) *Pseudomonas aeruginosa*
    d) *Proteus vulgaris*
    e) *Corynebacterium* spp
    f) Others
  2. Duration
    a) Acute (Fig. 5-3)
      (1) Clinical signs
        i) Usually unilateral
        ii) Mucopurulent exudate
        iii) Chemosis
        iv) Hyperemia
        v) Follicle formation
        vi) Pruritus—rare
      (2) Diagnosis
        i) Culture and sensitivity
        ii) Exfoliative cytology
          (*A*) Neutrophils predominate
          (*B*) Mononuclear cells rare
          (*C*) Many bacteria
          (*D*) Degenerative epithelial cells
      (3) Treatment
        i) Topical broad-spectrum antibiotics—combination of drugs (Table 2-5)
        ii) Protect with an Elizabethan collar or bucket if self-mutilation is a problem.
        iii) Remove encrustations and exudates.
          (*A*) Do this before medicating the eye.
          (*B*) Soak lids with warm water-saturated cotton.

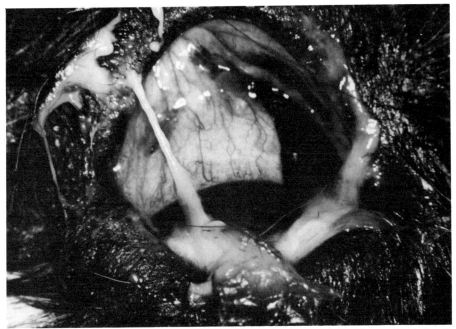

Fig. 5-4. Chronic purulent conjunctivitis in an aged female cocker spaniel, with associated chronic dermatitis. The lesions were bilateral.

           (4) Prognosis
               i) Excellent to good
              ii) Usually responds in 3 to 7 days
      b) Chronic
          (1) Clinical signs (Fig. 5-4).
               i) Often associated with other disease (e.g., atopy, lid defects, and ear infections)
              ii) Usually bilateral
             iii) Conjunctiva is thickened and appears velvety
             iv) Surface often appears dry and lusterless
              v) Follicle formation is prominent
             vi) Hyperemia
            vii) Swollen conjunctiva
          (2) Diagnosis
               i) Observe and identify the primary disease
              ii) Clinical signs
             iii) Exfoliative cytology (see Suggested Readings)
                 (*A*) Neutrophils predominate
                 (*B*) Many mononuclear cells
                 (*C*) Keratinized or degenerate epithelial cells
                 (*D*) Goblet cells

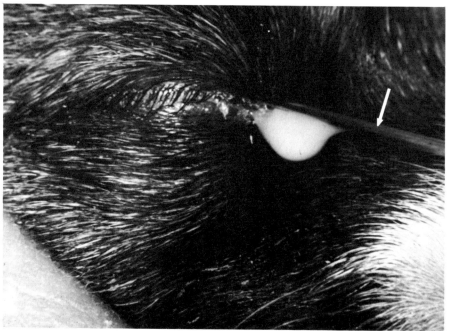

Fig. 5-5. Ophthalmia neonatorum in a basenji puppy, 6 days old. The puppy manifested bilateral elevations of the fused lids, accompanied by crying. The medial canthal region was separated carefully with a #11 BP blade and digital pressure. Arrow identifies the blade. Exudate is visible.

(E) Mucous and fibrin
(F) Bacteria may or may not be seen
(3) Treatment
    i) Similar to treatment for acute bacterial conjunctivitis
    ii) Antibiotic/steroid ointment is useful
    iii) Must identify and eliminate the primary lesion(s)
(4) Prognosis—guarded, with frequent exacerbations because it is associated with other diseases
c) Ophthalmia neonatorum (neonatal conjunctivitis) (Fig. 5-5)
    (1) Cause is usually *Staphylococcus* infection
    (2) Clinical signs
        i) Observed in puppies 1 to 2 weeks old
        ii) Lids are still fused and swollen due to exudate within the cul-de-sacs
        iii) May develop toward the cessation of ankyloblepaharon, and lids remain "glued" together
    (3) Diagnosis
        i) Clinical signs
        ii) Age
    (4) Treatment

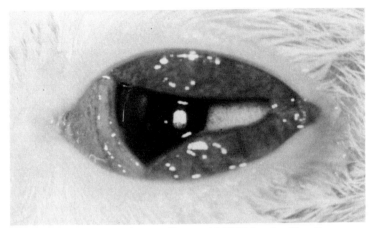

Fig. 5-6. Chlamydia conjunctivitis in a 1 1/2-year-old DSH female. The disease was unilateral without respiratory involvement. Intracytoplasmic inclusions compatible with *Chlamydia* were identified in the conjunctival epithelium.

   i) Lids must be opened, especially in puppies
      (A) Without proper drainage, the disease may involve the cornea and intraocular structures.
      (B) Opening should be done by digital pressure or surgical incision.
   ii) Antibiotics—topical Neosporin (Burroughs Wellcome) qid
   iii) Irrigation of the cul-de-sacs
   iv) Warm compresses
   (5) Prognosis
      i) Early diagnosis and proper therapy—excellent
      ii) Late—guarded to poor
B. Cats
   1. General
      a) Diagnosed more commonly in dogs than in cats
      b) May be due to the prevalence of viral infections in cats or lack of recognition of potential bacterial causes. The conjunctival flora in cats must be evaluated to increase the data base and the ability to diagnose conjunctival disease in cats. Bacteria were isolated from the conjunctiva in 91% of normal dogs. This must be recognized when interpreting culture results in dogs.
   2. Etiologies
      a) Chlamydia conjunctivitis (Fig. 5-6)
         (1) The agent of feline pneumonitis was previously called *Miyagawanell felis*, or psittacosis–lymphogranuloma–trachoma (PLT) group of viruses. It is now thought of as a

small obligate intracytoplasmic coccoid microorganism
closely resembling small bacteria, and definitely not a virus.
(2) Clinical signs
   i) Occurs in cats of all ages as an acute or chronic
      conjunctivitis
      (A) Acute
          (1) Usually unilateral
          (2) Chemosis
          (3) Hyperemia
          (4) Thick mucopurulent exudate
          (5) Follicles may be seen
          (6) May involve the opposite eye, if untreated
      (B) Chronic
          (1) Usually bilateral
          (2) Hyperemia
          (3) Thick, velvety conjunctiva
          (4) Occasional follicle
          (5) Symblepharon
              (a) Not specific for this disease—can occur as
                  a congenital lesion (p. 101)
              (b) A good history is important to eliminate
                  diagnostic errors.
              (c) Any condition that causes epithelial ex-
                  coriation can result in abnormal adhesions
                  of the conjunctiva.
   ii) May be endemic in catteries
   iii) Kittens born to infected or carrier animals
      (A) May manifest severe conjunctivitis when their eye-
          lids open
      (B) Some investigators believe this organism is the
          cause of ophthalmia neonatorum (see Suggested
          Readings)
(3) Diagnosis
   i) Clinical signs
   ii) Exfoliative cytology
      (A) Samples taken from palpebral conjunctiva
      (B) Stained
          (1) Any stain can be used
          (2) Giemsa stain preferred
      (C) Intracytoplasmic inclusions
          (1) Initial and elementary bodies in epithelial cells
          (2) Decrease as the disease becomes more chronic
      (D) Many polymorphonuclear cells (PMNs)
      (E) Few mononucleated cells
(4) Treatment

      i) Topical antibiotic ointments
        (A) Tetracycline—qid is my preference
        (B) Chloramphenicol qid
      ii) Chronic disease may require systemic administration of the above drugs
      iii) Steroids are contraindicated, in my opinion—the condition is worsened with the use of topical steroids; I strongly recommend against their use for this condition

    (5) Prognosis
        (A) Depends on duration of infection
        (B) Degree of involvement in the cattery
        (C) Immunity is short-lived, and reinfection is possible
        (D) Acute uncomplicated infections—good

b) Mycoplasmal (PPLO) conjunctivitis (see Suggested Readings)
    (1) Clinical signs
      i) Initially unilateral; may progress to the other eye
      ii) Conjunctiva usually pale, but may be hyperemic
      iii) Pseudodiphtheritic membrane—observed on membrana and can be removed without causing hemorrhage
      iv) Serous to mucopurulent exudate
      v) May be associated with upper respiratory infections caused by other agents (i.e., predisposed by stress)
    (2) Diagnosis
      i) Clinical signs
      ii) Culture—fastidious organism, requires specific media
      iii) Exfoliative cytology
        (A) Coccoid to coccobacillary clusters of organism on the epithelial cell wall
        (B) Exclusively PMNs
    (3) Treatment—topical ophthalmic ointments
      i) Tetracycline qid
      ii) Chloramphenicol qid
    (4) Prognosis—good to excellent

c) Salmonella conjunctivitis
    (1) *Salmonela typhimurium*—isolated from the inflamed conjunctiva of a cat that did not have intestinal disease
    (2) Increased suspicion for this pathogen in cats with conjunctivitis
    (3) Clinical signs
      i) Hyperemia
      ii) Epiphora
      iii) Blepharospasm
    (4) Diagnosis
      i) Culture
      ii) Exfoliative cytology

    (*A*) Absence of inclusion bodies or organisms on the cell wall

    (*B*) Many PMNs

   iii) Stool culture for *Salmonella* organisms

  (5) Treatment

   i) Must do a sensitivity study on isolate

   ii) Treat with specific antibiotic topically and systemically

  (6) Prognosis—in the absence of associated enteritis, the prognosis is excellent. Persons handling the cat should be aware of the potential zoonosis.

 II. Viral conjunctivitis

  A. Dogs

   1. General

    a) There are many systemic viral diseases that may affect the conjunctiva.

    b) Many gain entry through the conjunctiva but do not produce serious conjunctivitis.

    c) There is much more to learn about the viruses that may affect the conjunctiva as a primary target tissue.

    d) Many viruses that have been isolated from the conjunctiva are not pathogenic, and many that may be pathogenic have not been identified.

    e) Much research is necessary in this area.

   2. Adenovirus I (infectious canine hepatitis)

    a) Clinical signs

     (1) Early—ciliary flush

     (2) Mild chemosis

     (3) Hyperemia

     (4) Photophobia

     (5) Serous or seromucous exudate

    b) Diagnosis

     (1) Clinical signs

     (2) Immunization history

     (3) Exposure history

    c) Treatment (see p. 206—Uvea)

    d) Prognosis—good to guarded, depending on systemic disease

   3. Adenovirus II (infectious tracheobronchitis)

    a) Clinical signs

     (1) Bilateral

     (2) Severe hyperemia

     (3) Seromucous exudate

    b) Diagnosis

     (1) Clinical signs

     (2) Immunization history

     (3) Exposure

    c) Treatment
       (1) Treat the primary disease.
       (2) Give topical antibiotics tid to prevent secondary infection.
    d) Prognosis—usually good
4. Canine distemper
    a) Acute
       (1) Clinical signs other than systemic
          i) Severe erythema
          ii) Serous discharge
          iii) Blepharospasms
       (2) Diagnosis
          i) Clinical signs
          ii) Cytology—acute disease may demonstrate cytoplasmic inclusions
       (3) Treatment (see Chronic lesions)
       (4) Prognosis (see Chronic lesions)
    b) Chronic
       (1) Clinical signs other than systemic
          i) Bilateral thickened conjunctiva
          ii) Dry, dull cornea
          iii) Often thick purulent discharge
       (2) Diagnosis
          i) Clinical signs
          ii) Immunization history
          iii) Ophthalmoscopy
       (3) Treatment
          i) Topical antibiotics
          ii) Irrigation and removal of encrustations
          iii) Artificial tears
          iv) Therapy for systemic disease
       (4) Prognosis—depends on degree of systemic involvement
5. Other viruses
    a) Follicular conjunctivitis (Fig. 5-7)
       (1) Poorly defined disease
       (2) All other diseases must be eliminated
    b) Clinical signs
       (1) Severe erythema
       (2) Follicular hyperplasia
       (3) Moderate to severe blepharospasms
       (4) Serous ocular discharge
    c) Diagnosis
       (1) Eliminate other diseases
       (2) Clinical signs
       (3) Persistent lesions while treated with antibiotics
    d) Treatment

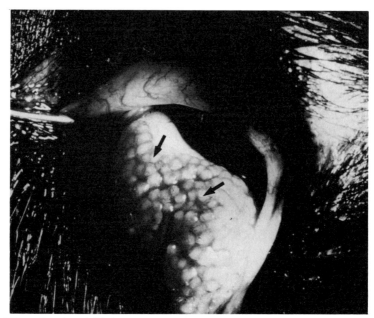

Fig. 5-7. Bilateral conjunctivitis in a 1-year-old male German shepherd. The third eyelid is everted, exposing the bulbar surface. Notice the "cobblestoning" due to lymphoid proliferation (arrow). These are solid, firm nodules, not vesicles. Etiology unknown.

(1) Treatment will change a chronic to an acute disease.
(2) Strictly palliative, at best.
(3) Topically anesthetize the conjunctiva or induce general anesthesia.
(4) Remove the follicles.
    i) Rub with a gauze sponge wrapped about the index finger.
    ii) Abrade with the back of a scalpel blade or other dull, *not sharp*, object.
    iii) Copper sulphate crystals
        (*A*) Astringent
        (*B*) Shrinks the follicles
        (*C*) Do not "burn" the surface
        (*D*) Method
            (*1*) Hold the crystal in a pair of thumb forceps.
            (*2*) Firmly but gently rub the crystal over the offending follicles.
            (*3*) Thoroughly irrigate the surface.
            (*4*) This usually results in marked inflammatory swelling—the owner should be forewarned or

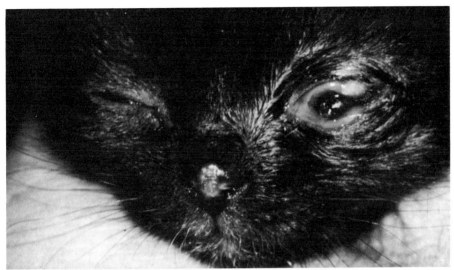

Fig. 5-8. Ophthalmia neonatorum in a 3-week old kitten. The entire litter was affected. The animals were successfully treated with IDU (Stoxil, Smith Kline & French) topically applied. Other anti-herpes agents are also effective.

       the animal kept in the hospital until the reaction is resolved.

  (5) Give antibiotic/steroid ointment following destruction of the follicles—q4h to q6h for the first 2 days, then tid until all signs abate

 e) Prognosis—guarded for this nondescript disease, until it is more adequately described and defined

B. Cats

 1. General

  a) More clearly identified in cats than in dogs

  b) Viruses that affect only the conjunctiva have not been identified.

  c) Viruses that infect the respiratory tract can be limited to the conjunctiva or in conjunction with respiratory tract infection.

 2. Feline herpesvirus I (rhinotracheitis)

  a) Three forms (see Suggested Readings)

   (1) Ophthalmia neonatorum—occurs in kittens 2 to 4 weeks old (Fig. 5-8)

    i) Usually, the entire litter is affected.

    ii) Ocular lesions are progressive and usually associated with a respiratory condition.

    iii) Mild, progressing to severe, blepharospasm

    iv) Subtle epiphora, progressing to a profuse mucopurulent discharge that results in "gluing" the lids together

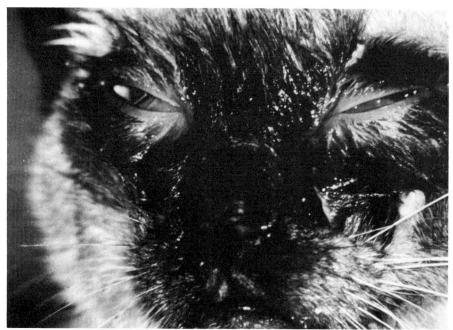

Fig. 5-9. Bilateral conjunctivitis in a 6-month-old Siamese cat. It was treated successfully with IDU (Stoxil, Smith Kline & French) topically applied.

      v) Mild conjunctival injection, progressing to severe chemosis, often with a pseudodiphtheritic membrane
      vi) Primary corneal lesions do not occur, but secondary ulcerative keratitis can be manifest.
      vii) Has a course of 10 to 14 days
   (2) Acute conjunctivitis—occurs in cats 1 to 6 months old (Fig. 5-9)
      i) Acute onset
      ii) Serous discharge with little or no purulent component
      iii) Conjunctival hyperemia but little or no chemosis
      iv) Concurrent upper respiratory infection
      v) Course of 10 to 14 days
   (3) Dendritic keratoconjunctivitis in older adult cats
      i) Mild conjunctivitis
      ii) Serous discharge
      iii) Dendritic ulceration (Fig. 5-10)
        (*A*) May be subtle
        (*B*) May require magnification to identify
      iv) Secondary interstitial keratitis may be observed.
      v) Blepharospasms
      vi) Course is variable and can be chronic.

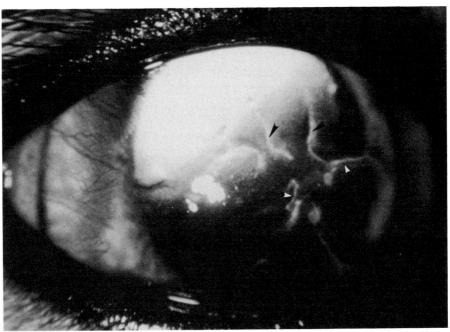

Fig. 5-10. Dendritic ulcerative keratitis (arrows) in an aged DSH with presumed herpes (rhino-tracheitis) virus. (Courtesy of Dr. Carol Szymanski, Ohio State University College of Veterinary Medicine.)

        vii) May be unilateral or bilateral
   b) Diagnosis
     (1) Age of the animal
     (2) Clinical signs
     (3) Virus isolation
        i) Specimens obtained from the conjunctival sacs placed in tissue culture medium
       ii) Inoculated on monolayers of feline kidney cells
     (4) Serologic tests
        i) Serum neutralization
       ii) Hemaglutination inhibition
     (5) Conjunctival and nasal smears
        i) Treated with fluorescein-conjugated herpesvirus antiserum
       ii) Examined with a fluorescent microscope
     (6) Response to therapy
        i) Although the above diagnostic tests are reliable and definitive, they are often not readily available.
       ii) the lesions described are ameliorated quickly by proper therapy; in my opinion, this provides diagnostic confirmation.

    c) Treatment
      (1) Antiviral (DNA) agents—available in solutions or ointments
         i) Idoxuridine IDU (Stoxil, Smith Kline & French; Herplex, Allergan)
         ii) Vidarabine (Vira-A, Parke–Davis)
         iii) Trifluridine (Viroptic, Burroughs Wellcome)
      (2) Available forms
         i) Ointments—administered q4h until clinical response is observed, then in decreasing frequency
         ii) Solutions—administered q2h until clinical response is observed, then in decreasing frequency
      (3) Immunization with live modified virus vaccine is prudent
    d) Prognosis—good in the absence of debilitating respiratory disease
  3. Calicivirus conjunctivitis (picornavirus)
    a) Clinical signs
      (1) Mild to moderate conjunctivitis
      (2) Epiphora—primarily serous exudate
      (3) Ulceration of the tongue and, less frequently, the nasal epithelium and lips
      (4) Relatively short course—7 to 10 days
    b) Diagnosis
      (1) Clinical signs
      (2) Tissue culture
      (3) Florescent antibody (FA) test
    c) Treatment
      (1) Prophylactic immunization is prudent
      (2) Symptomatic
         i) Topical antibiotics
         ii) Artificial tears
    d) Prognosis—good for uncomplicated conditions
  4. Reovirus—a very mild conjunctivitis
    a) Clinical signs
      (1) Epiphora
      (2) Serous discharge, which may progress to a mucopurulent one in more chronic disease
      (3) Respiratory signs usually absent
    b) Diagnosis
      (1) Clinical signs
      (2) Tissue culture
      (3) Serum neutralization test
      (4) Hemagglutination (HA) test
    c) Treatment—symptomatic—usually self-limiting
    d) Prognosis—excellent
III. Parasitic conjunctivitis

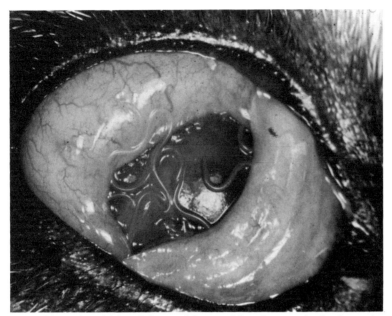

Fig. 5-11. Parasitic conjunctivitis (*Thelazia californensis*) in a German shepherd-type dog. (Courtesy Dr. Ralph Verheller, Whittier, California.)

A. General
   1. Observed in the eyes of several domestic and wild animals, as well as in humans (Fig. 5-11)
   2. Limited in distribution to California
B. Etiology
   1. *Thelazia californiensis*
   2. The life cycle has not been described, but an arthropod vector, the deer fly, has been incriminated.
C. Clinical signs
   1. Hyperemia
   2. Chemosis
   3. Serous discharge
   4. The worm
      a) 12 to 17 mm long
      b) Found within the conjunctival sac and behind the third eyelid
      c) Seen moving across the cornea
   5. Blepharospasm
D. Diagnosis—identify the worm within the cul-de-sacs
E. Treatment
   1. Administer topical cholinesterase inhibitor to kill the organism and facilitate manual removal.

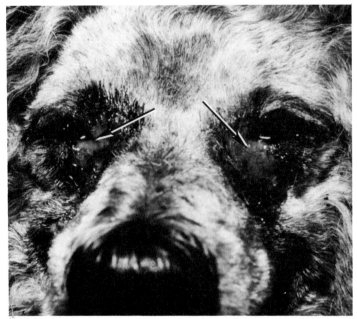

Fig. 5-12. Medial canthal erosion in an 8-year-old miniature poodle male. Erosion (arrows) presumed due to hypersensitivity to Staph antigens. *Staphylcoccus aureus* was isolated from lesions.

   a) Demecarium bromide 0.125% solution (Humorsol, Merck Sharp & Dohme)
   b) Echothiophate iodide 0.125% solution (Phospholine Iodide, Ayerst)
  2. Manually remove the worm with forceps and irrigate with saline.
  3. Treat the resulting conjunctivitis symptomatically.
 F. Prognosis—excellent
IV. Allergic conjunctivitis
 A. Etiology
  1. Many allergens
  2. Topical drugs—index of suspicion is high when an animal's eyes become worse while on medication
 B. Clinical signs
  1. Pruritis
  2. Erythema
  3. Hyperemia
  4. Serous to serosanguineous discharge
  5. May have severe blepharitis with excoriation (Fig. 5-12)
  6. May have inflammatory lesions
   a) Nasal cavity, nasolacrimal drainage apparatus, glossitis, and gingivitis for local allergens (see Figs. 4-12 and 4-13)

b) For other allergens the pharynx, gums, and ears may also be involved
C. Diagnosis
1. Exfoliative cytology
a) Eosinophils—few, but significant if present
b) Many PMNs
2. Clinical signs
3. History of exposure
D. Treatment
1. Identify and remove allergen(s).
2. Desensitization—Staph antigens
3. Give Naphcon Forte (Alcon) or Naphcon A (Alcon) tid or qid
E. Prognosis
1. Topical drug sensitivities—excellent
2. Other nonspecific allergens—guarded

TRAUMA

I. General
A. The conjunctiva is subject to direct and indirect traumatic injury.
B. Rarely is the conjunctiva injured without associated ocular damage.
C. The examiner should evaluate the entire eye when presented with a patient with conjunctival trauma.
II. Lacerations—usually the result of trauma or fights
A. Clinical signs
1. Chemosis
a) Minor—focal areas of swelling
b) Severe—diffuse edema, which may preclude an adequate examination of the underlying structures, cornea, or intraocular structures
c) May predispose to lagophthalmos and secondary drying
2. Observable tears in the conjunctiva—common in proptosis (see Chapter 3)
3. Exposed sclera dries and appears blue-black
4. Hemorrhage—variable
B. Diagnosis
1. History of trauma
2. Observable damage to the conjunctiva
C. Treatment
1. Simple lacerations—amenable to closure and heal rapidly
2. More extensive injury—treated according to the injury
a) Proptosis (see p. 53)
b) Examine all of the ocular structures and determine which periocular structures may be involved (e.g., orbital fractures)

3. Symptomatic therapy to accomodate secondary lesions
   a) Give antibiotic/steroid solutions if the conjunctiva is torn and the cornea is intact.
   b) Give antibiotic solutions if the cornea is ulcerated.
   c) Administer artificial tears to prevent drying.
D. Prognosis
   1. Simple, uncomplicated tears—excellent
   2. More involved injury—varies depending on the extent of the ocular damage
III. Subconjunctival hemorrhage
   A. Etiologies
      1. Trauma
         a) Automobile injury
         b) Animal fights
         c) Overzealous restraint
      2. Blood dyscrasias
   B. Clinical signs
      1. Overt hemorrhage visible under conjunctiva
         a) Focal
         b) Diffuse
         c) Color
            (1) Bright red—acute
            (2) Dull brown—chronic
      2. Uncomplicated hemorrhage does not cause subjective signs of pain.
   C. Diagnosis
      1. History
      2. Clinical signs
   D. Treatment
      1. Uncomplicated—no therapy needed; blood resorbs in approximately 2 weeks
      2. Complicated, particularly if anterior uveitis is manifest
         a) Atropine SO_4 1% to effect
         b) Antibiotic/steroid topical qid
   E. Prognosis
      1. Uncomplicated hemorrhage—excellent
      2. More extensive injury—guarded
IV. Conjunctival emphysema—usually associated with diseases of the paranasal sinuses as a sequel to trauma
   A. Clinical signs
      1. Presence of air subconjunctivally
      2. Usually secondary to overt head or chest trauma
      3. Hemorrhage may or may not be present
   B. Diagnosis
      1. History
      2. Clinical signs

C. Treatment—symptomatic therapy
D. Prognosis—usually excellent

CONJUNCTIVAL NEOPLASMS

I. Less common than neoplasms of the lids, but do occur and must be kept in mind
II. Conjunctival angiokeratomas—rare but reported in dogs (see Suggested Readings)
 A. Clinical signs
  1. Smooth conjunctival elevation
  2. Red or black
 B. Diagnosis
  1. Clinical signs
  2. Biopsy—discrete telangiectasias of the conjunctiva
 C. Treatment
  1. Surgical excision
   a) Close the lesion with 7-0 chromic gut.
   b) Provides specimen for histologic identification
  2. Cryosurgery
   a) Does not provide tissue for a diagnosis
   b) See Suggested Readings for technique
 D. Prognosis—good
III. Hemangioma and hemangiosarcoma—described in dogs
 A. Clinical signs
  1. Start as small telangiectatic blood-filled spaces
  2. Grow to a darkened enlargement
 B. Diagnosis
  1. Biopsy
  2. Histologic diagnosis
   a) Hemangioma—composed of endothelial-lined, blood-filled spaces
   b) Hemangiosarcoma—composed of solid sheets of endothelial cells lining small lumena that extend into adjacent tissue
 C. Treatment—surgical excision
 D. Prognosis
  1. Hemangioma—excellent
  2. Hemangiosarcoma—guarded
IV. Squamous cell papilloma
 A. Clinical signs
  1. Elevations at the limbus or caruncle
  2. Pedunculated or sessile
  3. May be hard or soft
  4. Variable color

a) Gray-red
b) Pigmented
B. Diagnosis
1. Clinical signs
2. Biopsy
3. Histologic diagnosis
C. Treatment—surgical excision
D. Prognosis—excellent
V. Squamous cell carcinoma
A. Clinical signs
1. Irregular elevations of variable size
2. White or pink
3. Frequently ulcerated
B. Diagnosis
1. Clinical signs
2. Biopsy
3. Histologic diagnosis
C. Treatment
1. Wide surgical excision
2. Cryotherapy
a) Rapid freeze ($-20°C$)
b) Slow thaw
3. High-frequency radio diathermy
D. Prognosis—good to guarded
VI. Papillomatosis (Fig. 5-13)
A. Clinical signs
1. Raised, irregular, sessile masses
2. Grayish-white
3. Variable sizes
4. May be found anywhere on the conjunctiva, cornea, or mucocutaneous junction of the eyelids
5. Considered a variant of canine oral papillomatopsis caused by
papovavirus
a) Oral papillomas occur in young dogs
b) Ocular papillomas have been reported in older dogs
c) May be a variant of the oral papovavirus or a completely different strain
B. Diagnosis
1. Clinical signs
2. Biopsy and histologic identification
C. Treatment
1. Excision
a) If the resulting lesion is extensive, close the defect with 7-0
chromic gut.

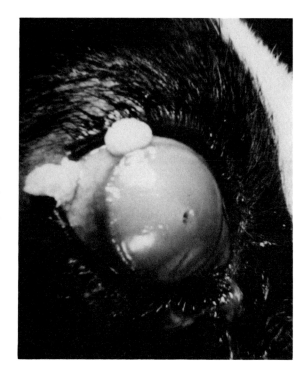

Fig. 5-13. Ocular papillomatosis with secondary keratitis and uveitis in a young Boston terrier. Central deep stromal ulceration and anterior uveitis presumed due to lagophthalmos asssociated with papillomas. (Courtesy Dr. William Jackson, Lakeland, Florida.)

        b) Treat the resulting defect as an uncomplicated conjunctival wound with broad-spectrum antibiotics.

    2. Cryosurgery

  D. Prognosis—excellent in the absence of other concommitant disease

VII. Benign epibulbar melanoma (melanocytoma) (Fig. 5-14)

  A. Clinical signs

    1. Dark-pigmented, smooth elevation on the conjunctival surface

    2. Usually observed near or at the limbus

    3. May be subconjunctival

    4. Usually nonpainful

  B. Diagnosis

    1. Clinical signs

    2. Biopsy and histologic examination

  C. Treatment

    1. Surgical extirpation—my preference

    2. Cryosurgery—efficacy is unknown

  D. Prognosis

    1. Superficial lesions—good to excellent

    2. Penetrating lesions to the sclera—guarded

VIII. Fibrous histiocytoma (see p. 184—Sclera)

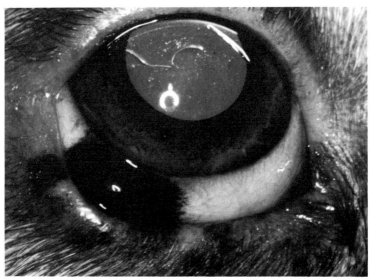

Fig. 5-14. Right eye of a 5-year-old Brittany spaniel female with benign epibulbar melanoma.

IX. Pseudotumor (iatrogenic granuloma)—repositol drugs may result in elevations of the conjunctiva that resemble neoplasms
   A. Clinical signs
      1. Whitish elevation with roughened edges
      2. Conjunctivitis—particularly perilesional
      3. Epiphora
   B. Diagnosis
      1. Clinical signs
      2. History of subconjunctival injection
      3. Biopsy
   C. Treatment
      1. Surgical extirpation
      2. Treat resulting lesion as described under Papilloma
   D. Prognosis—excellent

SUGGESTED READINGS

Bistner SI, Carlson JH, Shively JN, Scott FW: Ocular manifestations of feline herpesvirus infection. J Am Vet Med Assoc 159:1223, 1973

Buyukmihci N, Stannard AA: Canine conjunctival angiokeratomas. J Am Vet Med Assoc 178:1279, 1981

Cello RM: Clues to differential diagnosis of feline respiratory infections. J Am Vet Med Assoc 158:968, 1971

Lavach JD, Thrall MA, Benjamin MM, Severin GA: Cytology of normal and inflamed conjunctivas in dogs and cats. J Am Vet Med Assoc 170:722, 1977

Severin GA: Veterinary Ophthalmology Notes. 2nd. Ed. College of Veterinary Medicine, Colorado State University Press, Fort Collins, CO, 1976

6

Nictitating Membrane

ANATOMY AND PHYSIOLOGY

The nictitating membrane (third eyelid) has been considered by many an unnecessary structure of the eye of animals. That statement deserves an expeditious burial. The nictitating membrane is important as a protective structure, because it assists in spreading the precorneal film (possibly more important than the eyelids themselves in this regard) and covers the eye, protecting it from injury. Its gland produces approximately 50% of the lacrimal fluid and participates in the immune protective system of the eye, which provides a barrier against entry of infectious agents.

The membrana is located in the medial ventral aspect of the palpebral fissure and is covered by conjunctiva. It has a T-shaped cartilaginous skeleton that provides structural form and rigidity. This cartilage becomes very thin at the free lid margin and merges with the conjunctiva. This arrangement provides an extremely effective edge to spread the precorneal film. The base of the T extends ventrally and is embedded in the superficial gland of the third eyelid. This gland is a tubuloalveolar gland with multiple ducts located on the bulbar surface of the membrana. The gland extends higher on the bulbar side of the cartilage than on the palpebral side. The attachment of the conjunctiva to the bulbar side of the cartilage is very firm and difficult to separate. The bulbar conjunctival surface also is richly endowed with lymphoid tissue and can be observed on gross examination by everting the third eyelid.

The movement of the third eyelid is often described as passive forward displacement of the membrana when the eye is withdrawn into the orbit by the retractor bulbi muscle. This does occur, however, in the absence of globe retraction, animals, particularly cats, can prolapse the third eyelid. A third eyelid preparation has long been used in research to evaluate autonomic drugs. Strain gauges are applied to the edges and agents placed on the membrana, causing contraction or relaxation of the smooth muscle. Histologically smooth muscles are demonstrable in both cats and dogs. Horner's syndrome results in prolapse of the third eyelid; I believe that this prolapse is, in part, due to sympathetic denervation of these muscles.

Some investigators have suggested that a fascial retinaculum is present that secures the gland in its normal ventral position. I have dissected the third eyelid from many specimens and cannot identify this structure. Indeed, if such a structure were present, it would restrict the dorsolateral sweep of the third eyelid across the corneal surface. There is a portal, in the deeper aspects of the membrana, through which the inferior oblique muscle passes to insert into the lacrimal bone medially. This structure does not attach to the gland, but it

125

courses near its base. Further research is necessary to define more clearly this anatomic characteristic and its relationship to normal gland position.

DISEASES OF THE MEMBRANA NICTITANS

I. Congenital or inherited disease
    A. Protrusion of the nictitans gland (hypertrophy; cherry eye)—occurs only in dogs (Fig. 6-1) (see Table 4-1)
        1. Etiology—unknown, although there are several theories
        2. Clinical signs (see Fig. A-1)
            a) Reddened enlargement extending from the bulbar side of the third eyelid
            b) Mild irritation, little or no subjective signs of pain
            c) Epiphora
            d) Rarely, secondary corneal or conjunctival irritation present
        3. Diagnosis
            a) Clinical signs
            b) Breed predisposition (Table 4-1)
            c) Age of the dog
                (1) Usually occurs in dogs younger than 2 years
                (2) Enlargements in older dogs—consider neoplasia as a differential diagnosis
        4. Treatment
            a) Total excision is contraindicatcd.
            b) Partial excision has been advocated in the past and is still recommended by some.

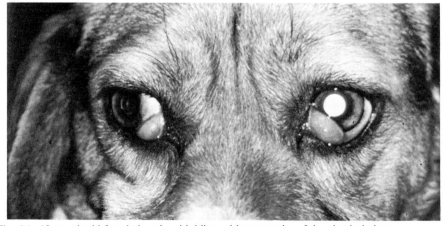

Fig. 6-1. 18-month-old female beagle with bilateral hypertrophy of the gland nictitans.

           (1) Only the portion that is prolapsed or hypertrophied is dissected free and excised.

           (2) This should be done only if replacement is not possible or if a differential diagnosis is necessary.

      c) Replacement therapy

           (1) I prefer Gross's modification of Blogg's technique, which requires general anesthesia.

           (2) Rotate the eye dorsally, with the third eyelid everted and exposed.

           (3) Make an incision perpendicular to the free lid margin, over the exposed prolapsed gland, extending to the limbus.

           (4) Carefully free the gland from the overlying conjunctiva by blunt dissection.

           (5) With a swedged-on spatula needle place two 5-0 chromic gut sutures into the gland at its most rostral prolapsed aspect.

             i) The bite should be parallel to the incision but medial and lateral to it.

             ii) The globe is rotated dorsally to expose the sclera.

             iii) The sutures are secured to the sclera by inserting the needle into the stroma, starting caudally and directed toward the limbus.

             iv) Both sutures are placed before either is tied.

           (6) Close the conjunctiva parallel to the limbus.

             i) This facilitates gland replacement.

             ii) 7-0 Chromic gut sutures are placed subconjunctivally to prevent corneal irritation.

   5. Prognosis

      a) When replaced—excellent

      b) When partially excised—good to poor (due to decreased tear production)

      c) When completely excised—guarded

           (1) Secondary keratoconjunctivitis sicca

           (2) Complete excision should be avoided at all costs.

           (3) The only justification for complete excision is neoplastic disease.

B. Eversion of the nictitating membrane (Fig. 6-2)

   1. Predisposed in giant breeds of dogs (see Table 4-1)

   2. Etiology—unknown

   3. Clinical signs

      a) Distorted third eyelid—prominent

           (1) The bulbar surface is exposed.

     • (2) The medial and lateral aspect of the free lid margin appear scrolled.

           (3) Usually not as red as prolapse, and often brownish in color

      b) Often bilateral, but can be unilateral

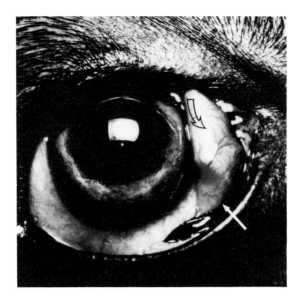

Fig. 6-2. 9-month-old male weimaraner with bilateral congenital eversion of the cartilage of the membrana nictitans. Free lid margin (small arrow). Bulbar surface of the third eyelid (large arrow).

   c) In severe disease, the gland may also be hypertrophied or prolapsed.
   d) Minor or no discomfort
   e) Minimal epiphora
   f) Minor conjunctivitis or, rarely, keratitis
4. Diagnosis
   a) Clinical signs
   b) Breed predisposition
5. Treatment
   a) Surgical intervention
     (1) Should be performed as soon as possible
     (2) I believe the condition becomes worse, never better, with time.
     (3) Usually observed in young animals
     (4) Method
       i) Anesthetize the animal.
       ii) Evert the third eyelid to expose the bulbar surface.
       iii) Make an incision perpendicular to the free lid margin and in the center of the everted or scrolled cartilage.
       iv) Carefully dissect the cartilage free from both surfaces of the membrana, without tearing the conjunctiva.
       v) Excise the distorted cartilage.
       vi) Closure is usually unnecessary.
6. Prognosis
   a) If corrected early—excellent
   b) If correction is delayed—guarded

          (1) Prolonged eversion produces a ram-horn effect on the medial and lateral tips of the cartilage

          (2) More complicated surgery is required to correct this defect.

C. Prominence of the membrana
1. Etiology
   a) Probably due to an enlarged orbit and an enophthalmic eye, in dogs
   b) Usually acquired in cats
      (1) Inflammatory disease of the peripheral sympathetic chain
      (2) Horner's syndrome (p. 49)
      (3) Nonspecific reaction to systemic disease accompanied by dehydration or cachexia
      (4) Patient must be critically evaluated when presented with acquired bilateral prominent membrana.
2. Clinical signs
   a) Bilateral protrusion of the membrana
   b) Conforms well to the convex surface of the globe, in contrast to cherry eye or congenital eversion
   c) Absence of hyperemia or conjunctivitis in uncomplicated condition
   d) Natural pigmentation alters appearance—the nonpigmented membrana is more obvious than pigmented membrane to the owner
   e) Cats may demonstrate signs of systemic illness.
3. Diagnosis
   a) Clinical signs
   b) Breed of dog
   c) History, particularly in cats
4. Treatment
   a) I do not advocate surgery for this condition
      (1) Some authorities recommend removing a portion of the prominent membrana for cosmetic purposes only in dogs.
      (2) The condition is a cosmetic defect and rarely causes significant sequela in dogs.
   b) In cats, systemic disease must be eliminated; then symptomatic therapy is warranted
      (1) Bilateral protrusion
         i) Self-limiting in about 3 weeks
         ii) Responds to low concentrations of epinephrine topically applied sid or bid
      (2) Horner's syndrome (p. 49)
5. Prognosis
   a) Dogs—poor for cosmesis
      (1) The condition is benign.

(2) The owner should be told that the condition is cosmetic rather than pathologic.
    b) Bilateral protrusion in cats
        (1) Uncomplicated—excellent
        (2) Associated with systemic disease—variable
 II. Inflammatory disease—diseases that affect the conjunctiva and lids also involve the membrana (see Diseases of the lids and conjunctiva)
III. Trauma to the membrana
    A. Etiologies
        1. Fights
        2. Direct blows
        3. Penetrating foreign bodies
        4. Surgical procedures
    B. Clinical signs
        1. Torn membrana
        2. Usually some hemorrhage—often the owner's complaint
        3. Swelling and chemosis
        4. Epiphora
        5. Some exudate, depending on duration of injury
    C. Diagnosis
        1. Clinical signs
        2. History
    D. Treatment—surgical repair
        1. Repair conjunctival tears.
        2. Place subconjunctivally sutures (7-0) chromic gut) so as not to irritate the corneal surface.
        3. For defects due to loss of tissue that cannot be reapposed:
            a) Mobilize the perilesional conjunctiva.
            b) Close the wound as in V-plasty (see p. 84).
    E. Prognosis
        1. Excellent to poor
        2. Depends on the extent of the injury
        3. Membrana can function event if scar retraction results.
        4. The tissues heal extremely well; preservation of the membrana is the objective.
 IV. Neoplasia
    A. Neoplasms that affect the conjunctiva can also affect the membrana (see p. 119—Conjunctiva)
    B. Plasmoma
        1. A poorly understood pseudoneoplasm observed in the third eyelids of German shepherds
        2. Clinical signs
            a) Early—erythema, progressing later to marked thickening and inflammation
            b) Irregular surface

       c) Usually bilateral

       d) Usually, but not always, associated with degenerative pannus

       e) Poorly responsive to therapy

    3. Diagnosis

       a) Clinical signs

       b) Histologic description

         (1) Predominately plasma cell infiltration

         (2) Some lymphocytes

         (3) Fewer PMNs

    4. Treatment—extremely resistent to therapy

       a) Topical steroids—q4h initially

       b) Systemic steroids—every other day or until controlled—0.5 to 1 mg/kg prednisilone

       c) Radiation therapy has been advocated, but I have had no acceptable response to this therapy.

       d) Chemotherapy and immunosupressive drugs have been unrewarding.

       e) Severe lesions resulting in secondary keratitis

         (1) Surgical extirpation

         (2) May be of transient benefit, not curative

    5. Prognosis—guarded and requires owner education at onset

C. Lymphosarcoma

    1. Observed in dogs and cats

    2. Because of the lymphatic tissue normally found within the membrana, it could be a primary site (this is conjecture).

    3. Clinical signs

       a) Gross enlargement—usually pink and not ulcerated

       b) The globe may be displaced.

       c) Epiphora

       d) Variable exudate

       e) Usually other areas of involvement, but I have observed lesions alone within the third eyelid of both cats and dogs

    4. Diagnosis

       a) Clinical signs

       b) Biopsy

    5. Treatment

       a) Generalized—chemotherapy (see Suggested Readings)

       b) Focal—surgical extirpation

    6. Prognosis—guarded

D. Squamous cell carcinoma

    1. Most common adnexal neoplasm, especially in white cats

    2. Eyelids are frequently involved

    3. The third eyelid may be involved secondarily by extension, but it can be a primary site.

    4. Clinical signs

       a) Gross enlargement

       b) Usually ulcerated and bleeding

       c) Rough surface

       d) Ears and lips are often involved in white cats

    5. Diagnosis

       a) Clinical signs

       b) Biopsy

    6. Treatment

       a) Massive surgical excision

       b) Radiation therapy

       c) Cryosurgery

    7. Prognosis—good to guarded, depending on the extent of the neoplasm

E. Other neoplasms—few confirmed reports, but should be considered when enlargements are observed

    1. Types

       a) Adenomas

       b) Adenocarcinomas

       c) Papillomas

       d) Mastocytomas

       e) Melanomas

       f) Fibromas

       g) Fibrosarcomas

       h) Neurofibromas

       i) Neurofibrosarcomas

       j) Hemangiomas

       k) Hemangiosarcomas

    2. Clinical signs

       a) Gross enlargements

       b) May displace the globe

       c) Secondary lesions are variable and are frequently the owner's complaint

    3. Diagnosis

       a) Clinical signs

       b) Biopsy

    4. Treatment

       a) Surgical excision, when possible

       b) Radiation therapy for radiosensitive neoplasms

       c) Cryosurgery

    5. Prognosis—good to poor, depending on neoplasm and extent

F. Miscellaneous enlargements

    1. Fibrous histiocytomas (see p. 184)

       a) Clinical signs

          (1) Frequently observed in collies, but other breeds can be affected

(2) Not reported in cats

(3) Fleshy masses, which most often involve the limbal region but have been observed in the lids and third eyelid

(4) Little subjective signs of discomfort, particularly early

b) Diagnosis

(1) Clinical signs

(2) Biopsy (see Ch. 8)

c) Treatment

(1) Many therapeutic regimens have been advocated (see Suggested Readings)

(2) Azathioprine—my choice

i) Obtain a baseline CBC to monitor bone marrow suppression.

ii) Begin the patient on 2 mg/kg/day for 2 to 3 weeks, then give 1 mg/kg/day for 2 to 3 weeks.

iii) Monitor the CBC for evidence of bone marrow suppression; decrease the dose accordingly.

iv) Continue to reduce the dose until the patient is no longer on therapy or the lesion begins to return.

v) Maintain the patient on the lowest possible dose for control (i.e., 1 mg/kg/week).

2. Membrana nictitans gland cyst

a) Clinical signs

(1) Enlarged third eyelid

(2) Possible displacement of the globe

(3) Epiphora or mucoid exudate

(4) Little subjective sign of pain

b) Diagnosis

(1) Clinical signs

(2) Excisional biopsy

c) Treatment—surgical excision

d) Prognosis—excellent

SUGGESTED READINGS

Gwin RM, Gelatt KN, Peiffer RL: Ophthalmic nodular fasciitis in the dog. J Am Vet Med Assoc 170:611, 1967

Latimer CA, Wyman M, Szymanski C, Winston SM: Azathioprine in the management of fibrous histiocytoma in two dogs. JAAHA 19:155, 1983

Theilen GH, Madewell BR: Veterinary Cancer Medicine. 1st Ed. Lea and Febiger, Philadelphia, 1979

7

The Lacrimal Apparatus

ANATOMY AND PHYSIOLOGY

The lacrimal apparatus is composed of the secretory, distributory, and drainage portions. (See p. 65 for a description of the distributory portion.)

Secretory Apparatus

Tears are the composite secretion of several glands. Lacrimal secretions have two components: basic tear and reflex tear secretions. To understand the clinical diseases associated with abnormal tear secretion, it is necessary to understand this complex physiologic function.

Basic Tears

The precorneal tear film contains protein (mucin), water (serous), and fat (lipid), respectively, from the epithelial surface out. These layers comprise the basic tears. The epithelium itself is hydrophobic; something must increase its wettability for the cornea to be kept moist and optically clear. This is accomplished by a protein (mucin) that interdigitates with the microvilli of the superficial epithelial cells and forms the first layer of the precorneal film. The intraepithelial conjunctival goblet cells produce mucin. They are found within the conjunctiva, most plentifully in the fornix, as well as in the conjunctiva covering the third eyelid. They proliferate in chronic conjunctival irritation, giving a thickened, velvety appearance to the conjunctiva and increasing the quantity of mucin, which is visible on gross examination. Chronic proliferative conjunctivitis may result in a decreased concentration of goblet cells as a result of metaplasia.

The second, and thickest, layer of the precorneal film is serous (water) secreted by the accessory lacrimal glands. These are Krause's glands and the glands of Wolfring, located in the fornix and at the base of the tarsal glands, respectively (Fig. 7-1).

The outermost layer of the precorneal film is a lipid layer, secreted by the tarsal (meibomian) glands, and possibly the glands of Zeis. The glands of Zeis are sebaceous glands at the base of the cilia, the ducts of which open into the follicle. The lipid layer prevents overflow of tears by increasing the tear surface tension at the lid interface. The precorneal film (basic tear) is secreted normally,

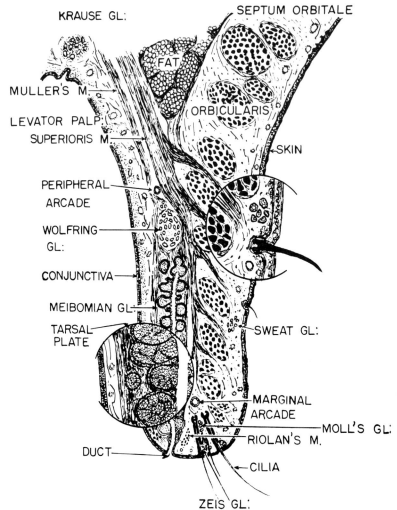

Fig. 7-1. Schematic drawing of cross section of the upper lid of the dog. (Prince JH, Diesem CD, Eglitis I, Ruskell GL: Anatomy and Histology of the Eye and Orbit in Domestic Animals. Charles C. Thomas, Springfield, Illinois, 1960, p.44.)

without stimulation. However, it alone is inadequate to prevent a clinically dry eye (see reflex tears).

The functions of the precorneal film are to: (1) lubricate the lids as they move over the cornea and conjunctival surface; (2) provide a medium for oxygen transfer to the cornea; (3) provide a vehicle for transfer of antibodies and inflammatory cells to the cornea; (4) provide an optically smooth surface on the cornea (as in polishing an optical lens); and (5) carry foreign material from the surface of the eye.

Reflex Tears

Reflex tears are produced by the lacrimal and nictitan glands in response to irritation of the cornea, conjunctiva, and lids. Psychic and olfactory stimuli also cause reflex tear production in humans. The afferent path for reflex tearing is the ophthalmic branch of the fifth (trigeminal) nerve to the brain stem. The efferent pathway is not well understood in animals, but branches of the facial, parasympathetic, and sympathetic fibers have been traced to both glands. Clinically, lacrimomimetic drugs such as pilocarpine increase tear production; this supports the hypothesis of parasympathetic innervation of the lacrimal and nictitan glands.

Clinically, tear production is measured by the Schirmer tear test. The test was first reported in 1903; it has been criticized in human medicine and modified to accommodate concerns. A Schirmer I, which measures reflex tears and is taken without topical anesthesia, and a Schirmer II, which measures basic tears and is taken after topical anesthesia, are used in human ophthalmology and by some veterinary ophthalmologists. Unanimity is lacking in human ophthalmology and inadequate information is available in veterinary ophthalmology to ascertain the value of the Schirmer II. The Schirmer I, on the other hand, is a valuable diagnostic test but too often overlooked. I advocate placing the strip in the lower cul-de-sac to the notch of the paper and closing the lids. This bends the paper in the proper place without handling and contaminating it with lipids or organisms from the operator's fingers. The paper is held in place for exactly 1 minute in the unanesthetized eye. The strip is removed and placed on the supplied rule and absorption is measured. For normal cats and dogs, the result is 15 mm or more in 1 minute (p. 142).

Drainage Apparatus

The openings to the nasolacrimal drainage apparatus are in the medial canthal area, at the mucocutaneous junction near the nasal termination of the tarsal glands. In contrast to the human puncta, dogs and cats have a slit-like rather than an elevated opening. This structure appears as an elongated pink slit in the pigmented conjunctiva. The puncta are continued as delicate tubules, called canaliculi, as described in Chapter 4. The canaliculi lie close to the conjunctival surface and course medially underneath the medial palpebral ligament, where they joint to form the lacrimal sac. The lacrimal sac is not as well developed in dogs and cats as in primates. It lies in the lacrimal fossa of the lacrimal bone. The nasolacrimal duct continues through the lacrimal canal of the lacrimal bone. The remaining portion courses in soft tissue to the nasal meatus. The duct often has defects between the end of the lacrimal canal and the root of the canine tooth. Clinically, this becomes important when determining patency of the system. For example, when the duct is irrigated, the patient may cough or sneeze during the procedure and have no fluid escape from the nares. The fluid enters the oral cavity or the turbinates, resulting in a gag or sneeze.

The distal openings of the ducts in dogs and cats are ventrolateral, near the margin of the alar fold. They can be observed by dilating the nares with a speculum. If necessary, they can be cannulated for retrograde irrigation of the drainage apparatus.

DISEASES OF THE NASOLACRIMAL APPARATUS

I. Inherited or congenital
  A. Imperforate puncta (see Table 4-1)
    1. Clinical signs
       a) Bilateral or unilateral epiphora
       b) Usually observed several weeks after weaning; may be due to decreased lacrimal function in puppies
       c) Presented for tear staining
       d) No subjective signs of pain
       e) Inability to locate and cannulate punctum
    2. Breed predispostion
       a) Cocker spaniel (American and English)
       b) Poodle (toy and miniature)
       c) Bedlington terrier
       d) Pekingese
       e) Miniature schnauzer
       f) Sealyham terrier
       g) Persian cats (relatively rare)—may involve cannuliculi and duct
    3. Diagnosis
       a) Clinical signs
       b) Observation of imperforate punctum—cannulation and irrigation of patent duct or normal punctum
          (1) Dorsal and/or ventral puncta may be imperforate; usually ventral
          (2) Irrigation causes ballooning of mucosa overlying atretic punctum
    4. Treatment
       a) Opening imperforate punctum
          (1) Irrigation defines the defect.
          (2) Incise or excise the conjunctival covering to reestablish the opening.
       b) Topical administration of antibiotic/steroid solution tid for 4 or 5 days is advisable after operation.
       c) When both puncta are imperforate, retrograde irrigation via the nasal meatus is necessary to identify them. They are opened as in (a), above.

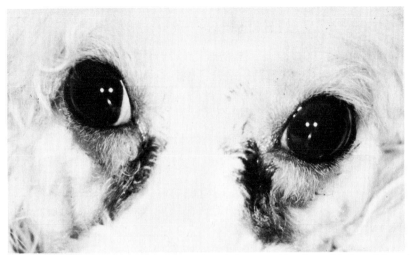

Fig. 7-2. 1 1/2-year-old white poodle with chronic epiphora resulting in unsightly staining of the medial canthi.

d) Persian cats may require a conjunctivorhinostomy (see Suggested Readings).
5. Prognosis
   a) Uncomplicated lesions—excellent
   b) Complete atresia, as in Persians—fair to poor
B. Epiphora of miniature breeds ("weepy dog" syndrome)
   1. Predisposed breeds
      a) Poodle—miniature and toy
      b) Maltese terrier
      c) Shih-Tzu
      d) Other toy terriers
   2. Etiologies
      a) Medial entropion
      b) Long caruncular hairs—act as a wick
      c) Trichiasis, distichiasis, or other conjunctival or corneal irritants
      d) Mechanical obstruction of the drainage apparatus, such as swelling or lid defects
      e) Inflammation of the nictitan gland—poor evidence to support this hypothesis
      f) Idiopathic—unfortunately, the most common category
   3. Clinical signs
      a) Tear staining—cosmetically unsightly brown or tan discoloration of the medial canthal area(s) (Fig. 7-2)
         (1) Bilateral or unilateral

  (2) Associated staining of other areas (i.e., the interdigital spaces, commissures of the lips, and around the genital orifices)
  (3) Those that do not have this staining characteristic should be critically evaluated for anatomic causes.
  b) Usually observed in puppies 2 to 3 months old
  c) Little or no subjective signs of pain
4. Diagnosis
  a) Clinical signs and owner's concern
  b) Fluorescein dye test
    (1) Hold the patient's head upward.
    (2) Fill the interpalpebral space with a solution of fluorescein.
    (3) Observe the external nares for presence of dye (should be obvious within 4 minutes).
      i) In my opinion, this is not a reliable test.
      ii) Approximately 30% of normal dogs have openings into the posterior pharynx and would have negative results to this test.
  c) Irrigate the nasolacrimal drainage apparatus.
    (1) Apply topical anesthetic.
    (2) Insert a blunt lacrimal cannula into the dorsal punctum.
    (3) Irrigate with warmed saline. The solution should exit the opposite punctum and the nares, or the animal will gag, swallow, or sneeze.
  d) Always examine for a potential cause of increased tearing or obstruction to flow.
5. Treatment
  a) Eliminate mechanical obstruction and/or irritation.
  b) Medical therapy
    (1) Poorly developed and obscure
    (2) Not for antimicrobial effect
    (3) May function to minimize pigments (porphyrin?) in tears and other secretions
    (4) Drugs advocated
      i) Oxytetracycline
        (A) 25 mg/day for a toy dog; no more than 50 mg/day for a 15-kg dog
        (B) Alternate 2 weeks on, 2 weeks off, or to effect
        (C) effective in approximately 80% of my patients
      ii) Metronidazole (Flagyl)
        (A) For dogs weighing up to 15 kg, 100 mg for 10 days
        (B) For dogs weighing more than 15 kg, 200 mg for 10 days
        (C) Has not been satisfactory in my experience
      iii) Conjunctivorhinostomy—see Suggested Readings)

            iv) Surgical removal of a portion of the gland—contrain-
               dicated, in my opinion
   6. Prognosis
     a) A very frustrating condition for the client
       (1) Educate the client.
       (2) Explain cosmetic versus pathologic condition.
     b) Research is necessary to identify more clearly the cause of the
        problem.
     c) The prognosis depends on the response to therapy and the ability
        to eliminate the cause
C. Ectopic lower punctum
   1. Poorly defined defect
     a) The punctum is located closer to the globe or several millimeters
        ventral to its normal position.
     b) This condition is said to be either primary or secondary to
        entropion.
     c) Because the upper punctum theoretically could remove tears, it
        is difficult to understand the etiopathogenesis.
     d) Further study and documentation are necessary.
   2. Clinical signs
     a) Epiphora of the involved side
     b) Abnormal placement of puncta
     c) Little or no discomfort
   3. Diagnosis
     a) Clinical signs
     b) Usually, a medial entropion
   4. Treatment—surgical correction of the defect (see Suggested
     Readings)
   5. Prognosis
     a) Ocular function—excellent
     b) Cosmesis—poor
D. Congenital alacrima (keratoconjunctivitis sicca; KCS) (see Table 4-1)
   1. Predisposed breeds
     a) West Highland white terrier
     b) Chihuahua
     c) Miniature schnauzer
     d) Miniature dachshund
     e) English bulldog
     f) Possibly others
   2. Etiologies
     a) May be inherited
     b) Congenital absence of the lacrimal and nictitan glands—
        hypothesis
       (1) Lack of development
       (2) Immune predisposition with subsequent degeneration

3. Clinical signs—all attributable to lack of tears and inability to blink
    a) Dry, lusterless cornea
    b) Corneal vascularization
    c) Thick, tenacious exudate
        (1) Gray appearance
        (2) When irrigated, it dissolves into a gray, thick solution
        (3) May prevent the lids from closing, causing lagophthalmus
        (4) Forms concretions on the lid margins
    d) Corneal ulceration—one or multifocal
    e) Thickened hyperemic, often pigmented conjunctivitis
    f) Palpebral fissure appears small
    g) Subjective signs of pain
    h) Secondary anterior uveitis
4. Diagnosis
    a) Clinical signs
    b) Schirmer I tear test—values:
        (1) Normal >15 mm/minute
        (2) Minor KCS, <15 and >10 mm/minute
        (3) Mild KCS, <10 and >5 mm/minute
        (4) Severe KCS, <5 and >1 mm/minute
        (5) Absolute KCS, <1 mm/minute
    c) Rose bengal dye test
        (1) Stains necrotic cells
        (2) Lacks specificity
        (3) Used in human medicine to detect very early KCS
        (4) Has little value in veterinary ophthalmology, in my opinion
5. Treatment
    a) Medical
        (1) The basic need is to supply artificial tears.
            i) Must be used frequently (i.e., q1h) for severe KCS
            ii) Solution or ointments may be used
        (2) Lacrimomimetic—pilocarpine
            i) Orally—in my opinion, too toxic and unnecessary
            ii) Topically—effective but can be irritating
        (3) Antibiotics
            i) In the absence of tears, the irrigating mechanism and possibly the immune defenses are compromised; therefore antibiotics are used to control the microbial flora.
            ii) Broad-spectrum, particularly for *Pseudomonas* and *Staphylococcous*
                (*A*) Gentamicin sulfate
                (*B*) Polymyxin B, neomycin, bacitracin
        (4) Mucolytic agent (acetylcysteine)—not used as an anticollagenase for this condition
        (5) Steroid

    i) Topical prednisilone acetate
      (A) Used as an ointment with a sulfa drug
      (B) Used morning and night
      (C) Should not be used at the same time solution is used—a minimum of 5 minutes between drugs is advised
    ii) Systemic steroids
      (A) More rational to use steroids in acquired KCS because of its potential immune etiology
      (B) Used early in the disease
      (C) Used as an immunosuppressive as well as an anti-inflammatory agent

(6) Combination of drugs to potentiate owner compliance (modified Severin's solution):

Adapt (Alcon/B.P.)	6 ml
Pilocarpine 1% or 2%	6 ml
Mucomyst-20 (Mead Johnson)	6 ml
Gentamicin for injection	2 ml
Total	20 ml

    i) I designate the solution according to the concentration of pilocarpine used in the mixture (i.e., solutions 1 and 2 are made with 1% and 2% pilocarpine, respectively).
    ii) The medication should be refrigerated, but it is irritating and, when cold, painful and the patient will resist it. Therefore:
      (A) Dispense a small medicine dropper bottle to be kept at room temperature.
      (B) Fill the small bottle daily with a 24-hour supply from a larger, refrigerated bottle.
    iii) Refrigerated, 20 ml will maintain potency for 1 month; potency and sterility may be compromised if more than 20 ml at a time is prepared.
    iv) Frequency of medication is determined by the severity of KCS.
    v) The patient must be reevaluated frequently to adjust the dosage.
    vi) Remove the most irritating components as the condition improves and replace them with equal volumes of Adapt (Alcon/B.P.) Listed in order of irritation.
      (A) Mucomyst-20 (Mead Johnson)
      (B) Pilocarpine
      (C) Continue until the only medication is Adapt

b) Surgical
   (1) When tear production is less than 2 mm/minute and medical therapy is ineffective, transposition of the parotid duct is an alternative.
   (2) This procedure is not a panacea and should not be presented as such.
   (3) Saliva is a substitute for tears, but it differs in pH and viscosity.
       i) May result in calcific deposits on the corneal surface
       ii) Runs down the face and frequently causes a moist facial dermatitis
       iii) Does not completely eliminate need for treatment, in most instances
   (4) The ability to salivate must be determined before operation
       i) Apply a drop of 1% atropine to index finger and rub some on the patient's gums.
       ii) Observe the punctum of the parotid duct in the mouth for presence of saliva. There should be a copious flow.
       iii) If saliva does not appear, surgery is not feasible.
   (5) Technique—see Suggested Readings
6. Prognosis
   a) Absolute KCS—guarded
   b) Severe KCS—guarded
   c) Moderate KCS—poor to fair
   d) Mild KCS—fair to good
   e) Minor KCS—good to excellent

II. Acquired
    A. Obstructions
       1. Puncta
          a) Etiologies
             (1) Inflammatory debris associated with:
                 i) Conjunctivitis
                 ii) Dacryocystitis
             (2) Foreign bodies—often accompanied by a mucopurulent exudate
                 i) Sand
                 ii) Plant material
                 iii) Plastic and metallic materials
          b) Clinical signs
             (1) Medial canthus may be swollen
             (2) Epiphora
             (3) Variable degrees of exudate
             (4) Associated signs of inflammation
             (5) Observation of foreign material
          c) Diagnosis

        (1) Clinical signs
        (2) Irrigate the nasolacrimal apparatus.
        (3) Demonstrate "casts" exiting the inferior punctum when irrigating.
        (4) Demonstrate foreign material within the puncta.
        (5) Negative fluorescein test—not completely reliable
    d) Treatment
        (1) Irrigate the nasolacrimal apparatus.
            i) Equipment
                (A) Topical anesthetic—proparacaine HCl
                (B) Lacrimal cannula—blunt 25- to 21-gauge
                (C) Optivisor or other magnification
                (D) Warm saline as an irrigant
            ii) Restraint
                (A) Tractible animal may be treated with topical anesthetic only.
                (B) An intractible animal may require a short-acting general anesthetic.
        (2) Manually remove plant material or other foreign bodies with forceps.
        (3) Treat the associated inflammatory disease.
            i) Culture the exudate and obtain sensitivity values.
            ii) Treat with appropriate antibiotic/steroid solution.
                (A) Give qid or more often
                (B) 5 to 7 days, or as improvement dictates
    e) Prognosis—excellent to good
  2. Canaliculi
    a) Etiologies—same as for puncta
    b) Clinical signs—same as for puncta, but foreign bodies are not usually observed
    c) Diagnosis—same as for puncta
    d) Treatment—same as for puncta
    e) Prognosis—same as for puncta
  3. Nasolacrimal sac
    a) Causes
        (1) Inflammation
            i) Chronic inflammation may result in obstruction of the lumen
            ii) May be secondary to conjunctivitis or the cause of conjunctivitis
        (2) Foreign material, as for puncta
        (3) Perisacular neoplasia or inflammatory lesions
    b) Clinical signs
        (1) Similar to those for puncta
        (2) Demonstrable swelling in medial canthus

           i) Usually painful

          ii) May erode through the skin when abscess formation is present

        iii) Pressure on the swelling results in exudate exiting either punctum

    (3) Usually present for chronic purulent conjunctivitis

    (4) Irrigation results in thick, tenacious material from opposite puncta

c) Diagnosis

    (1) Clinical signs

    (2) Dacryocystorhinography (see Suggested Readings)

d) Treatment

    (1) Irrigate the nasolacrimal system—usually requires general anesthesia.

    (2) Obtain a culture specimen in chronic conditions

        i) Culture

       ii) Sensitivity determinations

    (3) Place an indwelling catheter for chronic disease (Severin's technique)

        i) Pass a blunted nylon monofilament thread from the upper punctum through the system and out the nose.

       ii) Thread a PE 90 polyethelene tube over the nylon and pull it gently through to exit the nostril.

      iii) Remove the nylon thread, tie the two ends together, and suture to the face.

      iv) Allow the tube to remain for 2 to 3 weeks.

    (4) Medicate with appropriate antibiotic/steroid solutions

        i) Give medication qid or more often.

       ii) Decrease the frequency as improvement dictates.

      iii) Continue as long as the catheter is in situ.

    (5) Complete scarring and absence of patency

        i) This may occur as the result of:

           (A) Chronic inflammation

           (B) Allergic drug reactions

           (C) Postviral infections in cats

       ii) Conjunctivorhinostomy is the recommended treatment for this lesion (see Suggested Readings)

e) Prognosis—excellent to guarded, depending on the cause and damage

4. Nasolacrimal duct

a) Etiologies

    (1) Same as for puncta

    (2) Dental disease—may be revealed on examination of oral cavity

    (3) Periductular neoplasms

    b) Clinical signs
       (1) Same as for puncta
       (2) Dental disease
       (3) Deviated nose or swelling
    c) Diagnosis
       (1) Clinical signs
       (2) Skull radiographs
       (3) Dacryocystorhinography
       (4) Biopsy or cytology of exudate
    d) Treatment
       (1) Correct the associated lesion(s).
          i) Remove the offending tooth or teeth.
          ii) Biopsy and treat the neoplasm as indicated.
          iii) Dislodge and treat foreign bodies as for obstructed sac.
       (2) Conjunctivorhinostomy may be necessary if there is complete obstruction.
  B. Lacerations of the nasolacrimal drainage apparatus
    1. Regions involved
      a) Puncta—usually associated with torn medial canthus (uncommon)
      b) Canaliculi
       (1) Most common
       (2) Also occurs as a result of torn medial canthus
       (3) Etiologies
          i) Automobile accident
          ii) Bite or scratch wound
          iii) Flying object, etc.
       (4) Clinical signs—observe laceration and location
       (5) Diagnosis
          i) Made by inspection
          ii) Cannulation
       (6) Treatment
          i) Identify and suture both ends of the canaliculi
            (A) Cannulate the punctum and observe the cannula exiting the torn portion.
            (B) Cannulate the opposite punctum and inject dilute methylene blue to stain the distal end.
            (C) Grasp the distal end and cannulate it with a silastic tube for a distance of 6 cm.
            (B) Place tubing over the exposed cannula of the proximal piece and withdraw the cannula until it exits the punctum.
            (E) Suture the duct with 8-0 chromic cat gut.
          i) Close the skin as in a V-plasty (see p. 84).
          ii) Leave the tubing in place until the suture is removed.

          iv) Topically medicate with antibiotic/steroid solution tid or qid.

      (7) Prognosis—excellent

  c) Sac

      (1) Less common and usually results from similar but more severe trauma than lacerations of the canaliculi.

      (2) Clinical signs—similar to those for lacerations of the canaliculi

      (3) Diagnosis

          i) Observe the lesion.

          ii) Irrigate the system to determine the location and extent of the laceration.

          iii) Retrograde cannulation via the external nares may be necessary.

      (4) Treatment

          i) Similar to canaliculi repair, but usually more extensive

          ii) Identify the extent of damage and determine the feasibility of reestablishing the integrity of the sac.

              (A) If the laceration is easily identified, repair it as for lacerations of the canaliculi.

              (B) If the laceration is severe, the sac can be disregarded and a silastic tube placed antegrade and retrograde through the sac without closing the sac.

              (C) If the distal duct is obstructed, perform a modified dacryocystorhinostomy (see Suggested Readings).

          iii) Close the skin defect routinely.

          iv) Place an antibiotic/steroid solution on the eye qid for as long as necessary.

          v) Use additional systemic antibiotics at discretion.

      (5) Prognosis—same as for lacerations of the canaliculi

  d) Duct—trauma of this nature is severe and rare. The concepts of repair are similar to those for other lacerations, depending on the nature of the injury.

C. Inflammation of the nasolacrimal drainage apparatus—It is difficult to separate the areas of the drainage apparatus and therefore prudent to discuss the system only as it relates to the sac and to the duct

  1. Nasolacrimal sac—dacryocystitis

    a) Clinical signs

      (1) May be acute or chronic

      (2) Frequently observed as recurrent conjunctivitis

      (3) Often unilateral

      (4) Mucoid to mucopurulent exudate

      (5) Overt swelling of the medial canthus

        i) Pressure applied to the area results in exudate exiting the puncta

        ii) May erode, producing a fistula

        iii) Patient may exhibit pain on palpation

    (6) May cause an occlusion of the drainage apparatus (see p. 145—Obstruction of the sac)

  b) Diagnosis

    (1) Clinical signs

    (2) Irrigating the drainage apparatus

    (3) Culture the content of the sac

    (4) Dacryocystorhinography

  c) Treatment

    (1) Irrigate the drainage apparatus.

        i) Anesthetize the animal.

        ii) Place the cannula in the upper puncta and irrigate with warmed sterile saline.

        iii) Culture midstream exudate from the opposite punctum and make sensitivity determinations.

        iv) Advance the cannula to continue irrigating the remaining portion of the apparatus until it is void of exudate.

        v) Instill a broad-spectrum antibiotic solution.

    (2) Give antibiotic/steroid solution qid or more often for 7 to 10 days.

    (3) Give parenteral antibiotic.

    (4) Indwelling catheterization may be indicated for stubborn conditions.

  d) Prognosis—in the absence of a foreign body, excellent

2. Nasolacrimal duct

  a) Clinical signs

    (1) Similar to those for dacryocystitis

    (2) More often observed in animals with longer skull types than in brachycephalic animals

    (3) Epiphora is common.

    (4) Ocular exudate is variable.

      (A) Serous

      (B) Seromucoid

      (C) Mucopurulent

    (5) Conjunctivitis is as varied as the exudate

    (6) Dental or nasal disease may be evident

    (7) Obstruction due to atresia is possible in cats, but it has not been reported in dogs.

  b) Diagnosis

    (1) Clinical signs

    (2) Skull radiographs

(3) Dacryocystorhinography—most helpful
(4) Examine the mouth and teeth
  c) Treatment
    (1) Treat dental abcesses.
    (2) Assess and manage neoplastic diseases appropriately.
    (3) Treat atresia as for obstruction.
    (4) Treat uncomplicated inflammatory disease as dacryo-cystitis.
  d) Prognosis
    (1) Dental-associated disease—excellent to guarded
    (2) Inflammatory disease—excellent to good
    (3) Neoplastic disease—guarded to grave
D. Acquired hyposecretion (acquired KCS)
  1. Etiologies
    a) Iatrogenic
      (1) Drugs
        i) Sulphonamides
        ii) Phenazopyridine
        iii) Topical atropine, especially in cats
      (2) Surgery
        i) Removal of the nictitan gland for control of epiphora or correction of cherry eye
        ii) Removal of the lacrimal or nictitan glands for neoplastic conditions
    b) Systemic disease
      (1) Canine distemper
        i) Inclusion bodies have been demonstrated in the secretory glands of dogs with distemper.
        ii) The condition may be transient or permanent.
      (2) Upper respiratory diseases of cats that affect the conjunctiva
      (3) Any debilitating disease of dogs or cats
    c) Orbital or periorbital trauma
      (1) May result in neurologic KCS (proptosis)
      (2) Fifth or seventh nerve palsy
    d) Chronic conjunctival disease
      (1) May be due to mechanical obstruction of the ducts of the secretory organs
      (2) May be an extension of the inflammatory process involving the glands
      (3) May be due to alterations of the quality of the tear film or its components
    e) Autoimmune mechanisms
      (1) Concurrent disease indicative of underlying immunologic disorder has been reported.

      i) SLE

     ii) Rheumatoid arthritis

    iii) Pemphigus foliaceus

    iv) Atopy

     v) Hypothyroidism

    vi) Ulcerative stomatis

   vii) Ulcerative colitis

  viii) Glomerulonephritis

    ix) Chronic refractory pyoderma

(2) Histologic evidence—lymphocytic and plasmacytic infiltrates in 87% of lacrimal glands examined

(3) Specific and nonspecific autoantibodies

      i) Gammaglobulins have been shown to be elevated in dogs with KCS.

     ii) Rheumatoid factor and antinuclear antibodies are present in dogs with KCS

    iii) Antibodies to lacrimal and salivary ductules have been demonstrated in dogs with KCS.

f) Other causes of questionable validity

(1) Vitamin A deficiency

(2) Definitive (primary) neurologic origin

(3) Idiopathic—as more information is accumulated, this category will decline

2. Clinical signs, diagnosis, treatment, and prognosis—(see p. 141—Congenital alacrima)

E. Neoplastic diseases

1. Primary neoplasms of the lacrimal gland

a) Rare

b) Types reported

(1) Adenocarcinoma

(2) Adenoma

2. Primary neoplasms of the nictitan gland

a) Rare

b) Types reported

(1) Squamous cell carcinoma

(2) Adenocarcinoma

(3) Adenoma

(4) Hemangioma

(5) Mastocytoma

(6) Viral papilloma

(7) Fibroma

(8) Epithelioma

(9) Endothelioma

(10) Sarcoma

(11) Lipoma

           (12) Melanoma

      c) Clinical signs—see Neoplasms of the orbit

      d) Diagnosis

           (1) Clinical signs

           (2) Biopsy

      e) Treatment—tumor-specific

           (1) Surgical excision

           (2) Radiation therapy

           (3) Chemotherapy

      f) Prognosis—guarded to grave

  F. Cysts

    1. Lacrimal gland

      a) Reported in dogs

           (1) May be congenital or secondary to trauma

           (2) Definitive cause has not been determined

    2. Nictitan gland—see Chapter 6

      a) Reported in a dog

      b) Similar to lacrimal gland

    3. Clinical signs

      a) Cystic swelling adjacent to involved gland

      b) Usually painless

      c) May develop exposure conjunctivitis

    4. Diagnosis

      a) Clinical signs

      b) Surgical excision and histologic confirmation

    5. Treatment

      a) Must be excised

      b) Aspiration is only pallitive and will result in recurrence

    6. Prognosis—excellent

SUGGESTED READINGS

Covitz D, Hunziker J, Koch SA: Conjunctivorhinostomy: a surgical method of the control of epiphora in the dog and cat. J Am Vet Med Assoc 171:251, 1977

Gelatt KN (ed): Veterinary Ophthalmology. 1st Ed. Lea and Febiger, Philadelphia, 1981

Severin GA: Keratoconjunctivitis sicca. p. 407. In Agiurre GB (ed): Veterinary Clinics of North America. Vol. 3. WB Saunders, Philadelphia, 1973

Yakely WL, Alexander JE: Dacryocystorhinography in the dog. J Am Vet Med Assoc 159:1417, 1973

8

The Globe, Cornea, and Sclera

ANATOMY AND PHYSIOLOGY

The globe can be divided into three concentric tunics: (1) the outermost and largest, the fibrous tunic; (2) the middle, the vascular tunic; and (3) the innermost and smallest, the nervous tunic.

The fibrous tunic is composed of the cornea anteriorly and the sclera posteriorly. The cornea "fits" into the sclera as the crystal in a watch, with the sclera overlying the cornea at the transition zone or limbus. This anatomic characteristic prevents direct observation of the drainage angle of the anterior chamber. The limbus is of unequal width, being widest in the dorsal aspect from the 11 o'clock to the 2 o'clock positions. This makes the dorsal aspect of the iridocorneal angle the most difficult to examine with a gonioscope.

The horizontal diameter of the cornea is slightly greater (approximately 1 mm) than the vertical diameter. Many authors state that the cornea is thickest axially, but biomicroscopic examination demonstrates that the normal cornea of domestic animals and humans is thinner in the center than at the periphery. The diseased cornea may be thickened in any quadrant.

The cornea has four layers: (1) the epithelium and its basement membrane; (2) the stroma; (3) the posterior limiting (Descemet's) membrane; and (4) the endothelium. There is no evidence at this time to support the presence of Bowman's membrane, the second layer in the human cornea, in dogs and cats.

The epithelium is nonkeratinized, stratified squamous approximately 8 to 15 cells thick. The basal layer is columnar and firmly attached to the basement membrane by hemidesmosomes. This layer gives way to the wing cells, which become progressively more squamous, gradually losing their organelles as they move toward the surface. The surface layer possess microvilli, which interdigitate with the mucinous layer of the precorneal film. The entire epithelium is replaced every 7 days; this is important when treating superficial corneal diseases.

The stroma, which comprises 90% of the corneal thickness, is arranged in organized layers, called lamellae. The lamellae are composed of uniform diameter collagen fibrils with various acid mucopolysaccharides in the interfibrillar spaces. Keratocytes (corneal fibroblasts), found in the interlamellar spaces, form the stroma by producing the collagen that surrounds them. They also participate in the healing process. Lymphocytes, macrophages, and neutrophils are occasionally observed in the normal cornea.

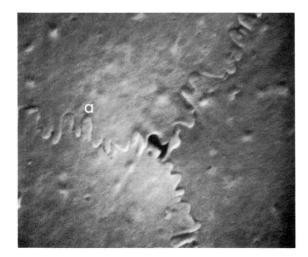

Fig. 8-1. Scanning electron micrograph of the normal dog's endothelium. a, undulating junction between two adjacent cells. ($\times 14{,}000$)

The organization of the lamella is, in part, responsible for the transparency of the cornea. Recently it was shown that the superficial one-third of the stroma is more reluent than the deeper two-thirds. Hypothetically, this is due to the parallelism of the lamella to the corneal surface in the deeper layers. It may also account for the increased superficial stromal relucency observed in early stromal edema.

The posterior limiting (Descemet's) membrane is the basement membrane of the endothelium. It is secreted by the endothelium and thickens with age. It is composed of fine collagenous elastic filaments, which allow it to bulge anteriorly in a descemetocele and to recoil when torn. Descemet's membrane is lipid-rich and does not stain with fluorescein in deep stromal ulceration.

The endothelial (mesothelial) layer is composed of a unicellular sheet of hexagonal cells, forming the anterior boundary of the anterior chamber. Adjacent cells interdigitate with each other (Fig. 8-1) and possess apical tight junctions. There is inconclusive evidence that they can replicate, but further research is necessary to document this property. Their ability to thin out and enlarge is well documented. The abundant organelles (mitochondria) found in the endothelial cells support their extreme metabolic activity. This layer acts as a mechanical barrier to fluid as well as a metabolic pump to remove water from the stromal layers.

Although the cornea is a metabolically active tissue, its transparency requires relative avascularity and acellularity. Other factors responsible for corneal transparency include corneal deturgescence (physiologic dehydration), regular arrangement of lamellae, presence of the precorneal film, and reflex tears, which provide irrigation to the surface by the lacrimal apparatus. The lack of keratinization and pigment results in a colorless transparent structure. The Embden–Meyerhof pathway, Kreb's cycle, and hexose monophosphate shunt are the metabolic pathways by which glucose metabolism provides the energy required for the avascular cornea. Oxygen is provided from the aqueous, atmosphere (via the precorneal film), perilimbal vessels, and conjunctival capillaries.

The maintenance of corneal deturgescence is complex and not completely understood. We recognize the endothelium and epithelium as important mechanical and functional barriers against stromal hydration. Active ionic transport across both structures and abundant Na–K ATPase levels in these structures has been demonstrated.

Overhydration of the cornea results in corneal cloudiness. This can be due to the separation and disarray of the lamella as well as to the presence of water. Transparency can be altered dramatically by applying pressure on the normal eye. This results in instant opacity, which clears when the pressure is released. This is explained by alterations of the lamellar arrangement.

The major portion of the fibrous tunic is the sclera, which has three layers. From the inside out, they are the lamina fusca, scleral stroma, and episclera.

The lamina fusca is a transition zone between the vascular tunic (choroid) and the sclera per se. It is composed of loose collagen bundles interspersed with uveal melanocytes and pigmented macrophages.

The scleral stroma consists of obliquely arranged, interlacing, variable-sized collagen fibrils with few fibroblasts. The stroma varies in thickness, being thickest around the optic nerve and in the area of the intrascleral plexus and thinnest at the equator and the lamina cribrosa. It also has several emissaria, through which vessels and nerves enter and exit the globe. The lamina cribrosa allows exit of the optic nerve through a sieve-like scleral aperture. The long posterior ciliary arteries and nerves lie superficial to the sclera in the horizontal plane, dividing the globe into a dorsal and ventral hemisphere. They perforate the sclera anterior to the equator. The short posterior ciliary arteries and nerves enter the globe perineuronally. The anterior ciliary arteries and vortex veins penetrate the sclera in the area overlying the ciliary body.

The episclera is a dense vascular layer that joins Tenon's capsule to the sclera. At the limbus, the conjunctiva, Tenon's capsule, and the episclera are blended together to join the sclera. The episcleral vessels participate in the inflammatory process of many diseases.

DISEASES OF THE CORNEA

I. General (nonspecific) characteristics of keratopathies (see Fig. A-1)
   A. Various degrees of pain, usually dependent on presence or absence of ulceration
      1. Superficial—usually painful
      2. Deep—less painful
      3. Nonulcerated—usually nonpainful
   B. Epiphora
   C. Loss of transparency (corneal opacities)

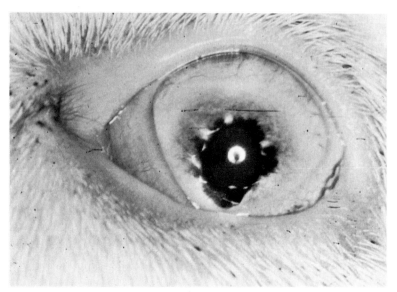

Fig. 8-2. Australian shepherd female puppy. Multiple ocular anomaly, including a small cornea (microcornea) in the left eye. Notice the notch-like defect in the iris (iridal coloboma).

      1. Edema
      2. Cellular infiltrates
      3. Pigmentation
      4. Scars
    D. Ulceration
    E. Corneal vascularization
      1. Deep—short and straight—originates from ciliary vessels
      2. Superficial—large and dichotomous
        a) Originates from conjunctival vessels
        b) Can form a halo around the lesion in 3 to 7 days
    F. Blepharospasm
    G. Exudates—type may indicate cause
    H. Axon reflex—corneal irritation may result in vasodilation of the anterior uveal vessels, causing:
      1. Iridocyclitis
      2. Aqueous flare
      3. Photophobia
  II. Congenital diseases
    A. Microcornea—small cornea in an otherwise normal eye (Fig. 8-2)
      1. Breed predisposition
        a) Australian shephard
        b) Collie
        c) Miniature and toy poodles

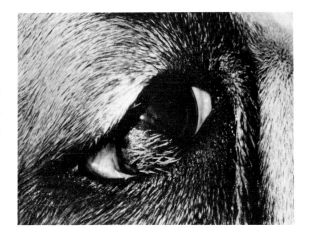

Fig. 8-3. Two-month-old male pug with a unilateral corneal dermoid. (Courtesy of Dr. Kerry Ketring, All Animal Eye Clinic, Cincinnati, Ohio.)

   d) Miniature schnauzer
   e) Old English sheepdog
   f) Saint Bernard
   g) Rare in all breeds of cats
  2. Clinical signs
   a) Small cornea (<12 mm)
   b) Often associated with multiple ocular defects
    (1) Microphthalmia
    (2) Goniodysgenesis
    (3) Persistent pupillary membrane
   c) More sclera visible
   d) In uncomplicated microcornea, sight is not impaired
  3. Diagnosis
   a) Clinical signs
   b) Measuring corneal diameters
  4. Treatment—none
  5. Prognosis
   a) Uncomplicated—excellent
   b) With multiple anomalies—poor
 B. Dermoid—see p. 100—Conjunctiva
  1. Clinical signs
   a) An ectopic island of skin on cornea (Fig. 8-3)
   b) Observed in dogs and cats when eyes are open
   c) Causes reactions similar to any irritant
  2. Diagnosis—by inspection
  3. Treatment
   a) Superficial keratectomy as soon as diagnosed
   b) The resulting lesion is treated as an uncomplicated superficial corneal ulceration
  4. Prognosis—excellent

    C. Infantile dystrophy (superficial opacity)
       1. Clinical signs
          a) Observed in puppies younger than 10 weeks
          b) Seen as noninflammatory superficial opacities
          c) No other demonstrable or associated lesions
       2. Diagnosis—by observation
       3. Treatment—none is necessary
       4. Prognosis—excellent—clears spontaneously
    D. Persistent pupillary membrane (PPM) (see Table 4-1)
       1. Breed predisposition
          a) Most prevalent in basenjis and considered inherited in this breed
             (see Suggested Readings)
          b) Seen in other dogs; cause unknown
          c) Rarely seen in cats
       2. Clinical signs
          a) Secondary lesions
             (1) Corneal opacity when inserted into endothelium
             (2) Cataracts when attached to lens capsule
          b) May bridge the pupil
          c) Originate from the iris collarette, which distinguishes them from
             inflammatory strands—most important diagnostic clue
       3. Diagnosis—by observation
       4. Treatment—none recommended
       5. Prognosis—owner should be informed of potential inheritance in
         dogs
          a) Uncomplicated—excellent
          b) Secondary lesions
             (1) Severe corneal opacity—guarded
             (2) Severe lens opacity—guarded
III. Acquired diseases of the cornea
    A. Superficial keratitis with ulceration—limited to epithelium and anterior
       stromal layers
       1. Simple ulcerative keratitis
          a) Etiology
             (1) Trauma—mechanical
                i) Lid defects—entropion, ectropion, etc.
                ii) Ectopic cilium, trichiasis, etc.
                iii) Foreign bodies under third eyelid (Fig. 8-4)
             (2) Chemical
             (3) Infection after superficial injury
          b) Clinical signs
             (1) Variable size
             (2) No tendency to spread or perforate if uncomplicated
             (3) Photophobia—usually severe
             (4) Blepharospasm

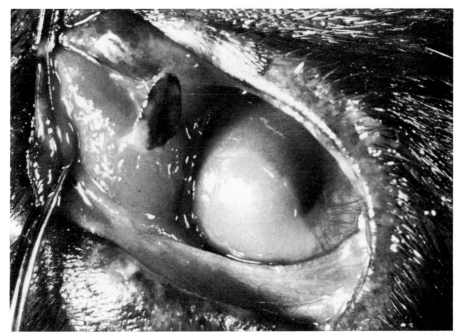

Fig. 8-4. Four-year-old German shepherd-type female with a plant foreign body under the third eyelid. The ulcerated keratitis healed uneventfully once the plant material was removed.

        (5) Epiphora
        (6) Pain
        (7) Little or no cellular infiltration or edema early
        (8) Fluorescein positive
    c) Diagnosis
        (1) By observation
        (2) Evert lids and examine for cilia and foreign bodies, etc. (Fig. 8-4)
        (3) Clinical signs
    d) Treatment
        (1) Remove the inciting cause
        (2) When signs of anterior uveitis are present, use atropine SO_4 1% to effect
        (3) Antibiotics—tid or more
          i) Usually prophylactic
          ii) Therapeutic, if associated with an infectious agent(s)
            (A) Specific antibiotic if known
            (B) Broad-spectrum antibiotic if unknown
                (1) Gentamicin ointment
                (2) Neosporin ointment (Burroughs Wellcome)

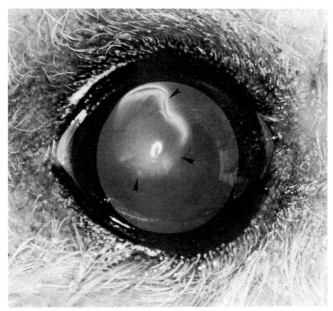

Fig. 8-5. Eight-year-old poodle with an indolent-like ulcer in the left eye. Arrows outline the redundant border.

    e) Prognosis—uncomplicated—excellent

2. Indolent ulcer (refractory, benign, rodent, boxer ulcer, epithelial erosion) (Fig. 8-5)

    a) Etiology—unknown

        (1) Virus—never isolated

        (2) Neurotrophic—never proven

        (3) Basement membrane dystrophy—in my opinion, hemidesmosomes are poorly attached to the basement membrane

    b) Breed predisposition (see Table 4-1)

    c) Age

        (1) Most frequently in mature adults

        (2) Seldom in dogs younger than 1 year

    d) Clinical signs

        (1) Little or no subjective sign of pain

        (2) Mild epiphora

        (3) Mild blepharospasm

        (4) Little or no corneal edema

        (5) Central or paracentral shallow ulcer, fluorescein-positive

        (6) Overhanging (redundant) border—important characteristic

        (7) May spread across initially affected eye; may also involve opposite eye

        (8) No tendency to penetrate or perforate when uncomplicated

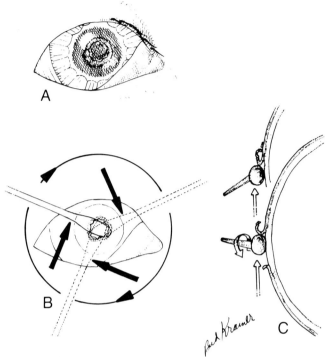

Fig. 8-6. Schematic drawing, demonstrating technique of abrading loose epithelium. (A) Gross appearance, demonstrating loose, redundant border. (B) Method of moving 360° around the ulceration. (C) Demonstration of direction to roll the dry sterile cotton applicator to effect removal of redundant epithelial margin.

(9) No sex predisposition, in my practice

e) Diagnosis
  (1) Clinical signs—particularly the absence of significant pain and the redundant border
  (2) Eliminate other possible causes

f) Treatment
  (1) Remove the redundant border to normal epithelial tissue (Fig. 8-6).
    i) Anesthetize the eye, or the animal if necessary.
    ii) Remove the border with a sterile dry cotton applicator with gentle but firm outward pressure on the loose epithelium.
    iii) Continue until the remaining epithelium is firmly attached.
  (2) Stain the eye and record the size of the resulting lesion.
  (3) Reevaluate the eye in 72 hours and observe for decrease in size.

      i) Compare with the record.

      ii) Should be smaller, preferably one-half the previous size.

      iii) *Do not* remove new epithelium if the lesion is decreasing adequately—the epithelium in any healing ulcers, including this type of ulcer, is poorly attached for as long as 6 weeks.

      iv) If the lesion is no smaller than the initial postdebridement ulcer, repeat the debriding procedure.

(4) Protective bandages—optional—may be necessary for 2 or 3 weeks

      i) Third eyelid flap

      ii) Soft contact lenses

(5) Broad-spectrum antibiotics—prophylactic only—Neosporin (Burroughs Wellcome) bid or tid daily

(6) Mydriatic—used only if signs of anterior uveitis are present—atropine SO_4 1% to effect

(7) Steroids are contraindicated until epithelization occurs; then antibiotic/steroid ointments are substituted for antibiotics

(8) Reproductive hormones have not proven effective in my experience

  g) Prognosis

    (1) For sight—good to excellent

    (2) Healing may be extremely slow.

      i) The owner should be informed that the eye may get worse before it gets better.

      ii) Complete healing in some patients has taken 3 months in my practice.

      iii) Severe scars may result if secondary problems arise.

    (3) Healing may also be rapid and uneventful.

    (4) There is a tendency for recurrence in either eye.

    (5) Owner education and explanation of the problem are the most important parts of successful management.

3. Dendritic (serpent) ulcers

  a) Etiologies

    (1) Canine infectious distemper—questionable cause, in my opinion

      i) Ulceration may be directly associated with destruction of epithelium.

      ii) Ulceration may be secondary to acute dacryoadenitis and exposure.

    (2) Feline rhinotracheitis (see p. 111—Conjunctiva)

      i) Older cats

      ii) The only confirmed cause of dendritic ulcer in small animals

  b) Clinical signs

(1) Ulcerations—acute or chronic
    i) May spread and branch along course of the corneal sensory nerves
    ii) Complications may predispose to perforation—very rare
      (A) Secondary infection
      (B) Autolytic reaction (see p.165—Collagenase ulcer)
(2) Exudate
    i) Serous (early)—usually virus-induced
    ii) Purulent—usually secondary bacterial component
    iii) May be thick and tenacious if tear production is diminished or absent
(3) Blepharospasm (pain)
(4) Epiphora
(5) Associated conjunctivitis
(6) Photophobia
(7) Iritis—may produce hypopyon (see p.197—Anterior uveitis)
c) Diagnosis
  (1) Clinical signs
  (2) Virus isolation
  (3) Rising antibody titers
  (4) Immunofluorescent cytology
  (5) Electron microscopic examination to identify viral particles
  (6) Response to therapy—my preference
d) Treatment
  (1) Directed toward specific disease—rhinotracheitis (herpes) virus
    i) Idoxuridine (IDU)—0.1% solution q2h; 0.5% ointment q4h
    ii) Trifluridine 1% solution q2h
    iii) Adenine arabinoside 3% ointment q4h
  (2) Symptomatic therapy for keratitis
    i) Antibiotics
      (A) Broad-spectrum
      (B) Specific if culture and sensitivity tests have been performed
    ii) Mydriatics
    iii) Artificial tears
    iv) Collyria—should be used prior to instillation of medicaments
      (A) Purulent or tenacious exudative lesions decrease efficacy of drugs.
      (B) Collyria should be warmed.
e) Prognosis
  (1) Uncomplicated herpes—excellent
  (2) Complicated distemper-associated keratitis—guarded

4. Mycotic keratitis—extremely rare in dogs and cats
    a) Etiologies
        (1) Specific fungi
            i) Candidiasis
            ii) *Aspergillosis*
            iii) Rhinosporidiosis
            iv) Others
        (2) Predisposition
            i) Chronic use of topical antibiotic/steroids
            ii) Perforating or traumatic injury with contamination
    b) Clinical signs
        (1) Chronic nonresponsive keratitis
        (2) Corneal involvement may help to identify agent
            i) *Candidiasis*—raised plaque-like calcific lesions sur-
                rounded by ulceration
            ii) Aspergillosis—severe keratomalacia
            iii) Rhinosporidiosis—multifocal paracentral superficial
                opacities that are relatively painless
        (3) Epiphora
        (4) Blepharospasm
        (5) Deep and superficial corneal vascularization
        (6) Ciliary injection
        (7) Hypopyon
        (8) Lesions associated with keratomalacia may perforate (see p.
            165—Deep stromal ulceration)
    c) Diagnosis
        (1) Clinical signs
        (2) Cytologic study—quickest and easiest
        (3) Culture
    d) Treatment
        (1) Lesions with plaque formation or keratomalcia
            i) Superficial keratectomy—used for culture, cytology,
                and histopathology in addition to removing abnormal tis-
                sue or debris
            ii) Cauterization—should be used with caution
                (A) Trichloracetic acid (TCA)—severe cauterant; de-
                    stroys surface protein as well as fungi
                (B) 7% tincture of iodine—excellent antiseptic and
                    anticollagenase
            iii) Antifungal agents (see p. 19—Pharmacology)
            iv) Conjunctival flap for severe malatic disease
        (2) Some lesions have been reported as self-limiting
            (rhinosporidiosis).
    e) Prognosis

       (1) Excellent to grave, depending on agent and degree of involvement

       (2) May require several weeks or months to heal

  5. Neuroparalytic keratitis

    a) Etiologies—lesions of the trigeminal (fifth) nerve or ganglion (rare)

      (1) Infection

      (2) Trauma (i.e., proptosis)

    b) Clinical signs

      (1) Insensitive cornea

      (2) Exposure keratitis

      (3) Ulceration

      (4) Dry, lusterless cornea

      (5) Mimics KCS

    c) Diagnosis

      (1) Clinical signs

      (2) History

      (3) Demonstration of corneal insensitivity

    d) Treatment

      (1) Determine and treat inciting etiology

      (2) Artificial tears

      (3) Antibiotics

      (4) Protective permanent tarsorrhaphy

      (5) Enucleation

    e) Prognosis—due to difficulty in determining a specific etiology, the condition carries a grave prognosis for recovery

B. Deep stromal ulceration (to Descemet's membrane) (Fig. 8-7)

  1. Etiologies

    a) Corneal malacia and lysis (collagenase ulceration)

      (1) Inciting agents

        i) *Pseudomonas* and other bacteria

        ii) Fungus

        iii) Alkaline agents and burns

      (2) Enzymes

        i) Protease—secreted by many organisms

        ii) Collagenase

          (*A*) Released from necrotizing corneal cells

          (*B*) Self-perpetuating, even in the absence of exciting infectious agent

    b) Traumatic

    c) Exposure keratitis

      (1) Prominent-eyed breeds

      (2) Ectropion

      (3) Buphthalmos

      (4) Lagophthalmos

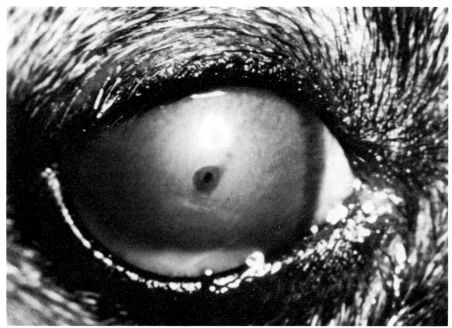

Fig. 8-7. Terrier-type 3-year-old female with an acute primary deep corneal ulcer (descemetocele) and secondary anterior uveitis predisposing to hypopyon.

  2. Clinical signs
     a) Keratomalacia—inflammation, hydropic degeneration, and necrosis due to proteolytic enzymes (see p. 165—corneal malacia and lysis)
       (1) Hazy cornea, which appears to "melt"
       (2) Corneal infiltration
       (3) Corneal vascularization
          i) Deep—short, brush-like
          ii) Superficial—dichotomous
     b) Pain
       (1) Deeper lesions—less painful
       (2) Superficial lesions—very painful
     c) *Pseudomonas* ulcers (Figs. 8-7 and 8-8)
       (1) Have a tendency to penetrate but do not spread circumferentially
       (2) Can penetrate to Descemet's membrane within 24 hours
     d) Corneal opacity—variable
     e) Exudate—usually purulent
     f) Blepharospasms
     g) Anterior uveitis
       (1) Flare
       (2) Photophobia

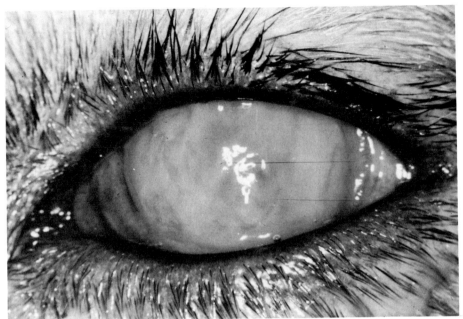

Fig. 8-8. Nine-month-old beagle male with experimentally induced *Pseudomonas* ulcerative keratitis with marked keratomalacia.

    (3) Swollen iris

    (4) Hypopyon—usually sterile

    (5) Hypotony

  3. Diagnosis

    a) Clinical signs

    b) Rapid progression of the ulcer

    c) Cytology, culture, or histopathology

  4. Treatment—determine the cause and treat it specifically

    a) Antifungal

    b) Antibiotics—should be effective against *Pseudomonas*

      (1) Topical

      (2) Systemic

    c) Anticollagenase drugs

      (1) Acetylcysteine 20% in equal parts of Adapt (Alcon/B.P.) qid—refrigerate

      (2) Penicillamine

    d) Mydriatic/cycloplegic agents—Atropine SO_4 1% to effect

    e) Antiprostaglandins—systemically

    f) Surgery

      (1) Conjunctival flap

  (2) Corneal, scleral, conjunctival transposition (see Suggested Readings)

  (3) Permanent medial and/or lateral tarsorrhaphy to correct lagophthalmos

 g) Prognosis—grave to good, depending on degree of corneal and uveal involvement

C. Superficial keratitis without ulceration (see Fig. A-1)

 1. Degenerative pannus (chronic superficial keratitis, Uberreiter's syndrome) (Fig. 8-9) (see Table 4-1)

  a) Etiologies—essentially unknown

   (1) Familial predisposition

   (2) Cell-mediated immunity to corneal and uveal antigens

   (3) Environmental enhancement (i.e., ultraviolet light)

  b) Breed predisposition (see Table 4-1)

  c) Clinical signs

   (1) Definition describes some of the signs—subepithelial proliferation with vascularization and accompanying pigmentation

   (2) Age—usually older than 1-1/2 years

   (3) Cornea has a "meaty" appearance

   (4) Little or no pain

   (5) Usually bilateral, but not necessarily symmetric

   (6) Usually starts at the lateral limbus, but can start anywhere

   (7) Progresses across cornea, ultimately causing blindness

    i) The leading margin may be cloudy due to separation of the corneal lamella.

    ii) The leading margin may demonstrate a dystrophic-like lesion.

   (8) Owners may complain of dog being exposed to a cat or neighbor who "attacked" it

   (9) Infiltration of third eyelid with plasma cells and lymphocytes (plasmoma) (p. 130)

  d) Diagnosis

   (1) Clinical signs—most important

   (2) Absence of any demonstrable cause (e.g., mechanical irritation)

   (3) Predisposed breeds

  e) Treatment

   (1) Directed toward the apparent immune-mediated predisposition

    i) Prednisilone acetate/sulfa ointment—my preference

     (A) Obtain an adequate level in the superficial structures.

     (B) Start q4h for the first week (see Fig. 8-9A).

     (C) Give q6h for the second week.

     (D) Give q8h for the third week.

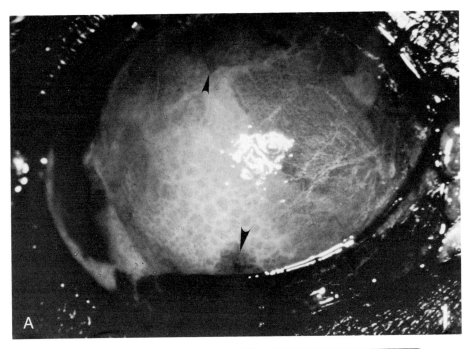

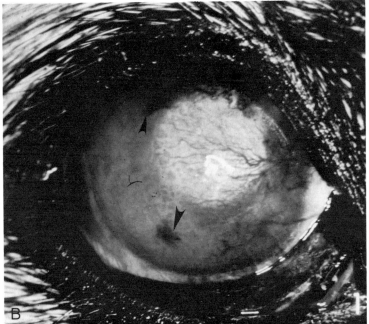

Fig. 8-9. (A) Six-year-old female German shepherd with advanced degenerative pannus before treatment. The eyes appeared red, and the dog was clinically blind. (B) Six days after topical medication alone had begun. Tapetal reflection is visible. Arrows identify the same pigmented spots in both figures for orientation.

(E) Give q12h for the fourth week.

(F) Continue to decrease at weekly intervals until lesion starts to return, then return to controlled frequency.

ii) Subconjunctival injections—not a panacea and not necessary in most instances

(2) Alternative therapy—not applicable, in my opinion

i) Cautery—chemical keratectomy

ii) Superficial keratectomy—not curative and removes stroma

iii) Beta radiation—predisposes to bullous keratitis 12 to 18 months after therapy

f) Prognosis

(1) Client education is important for client satisfaction.

i) Animal must be maintained on therapy for the rest of its life.

ii) Periodic (once or twice per year) reevaluation is necessary.

(2) Control—excellent

(3) Cure—grave

2. Pannus—other than degenerative (pigmentary keratitis; melanosis oculi)

a) Etiologies

(1) Chronic irritation—many causes

(2) Sequella to surgery or trauma

(3) Sequella to absolute glaucoma

b) Clinical signs

(1) Similar to those for degenerative pannus but adjacent to irritative lesion(s)

(2) The predisposing etiology usually can be identified.

i) Entropion

ii) Chronic conjunctivitis

iii) Ectropion

iv) KCS

v) Lagophthalmos

(3) Frequently bilateral, but can be unilateral

(4) Overt signs of the inciting disease may be present.

c) Diagnosis

(1) Clinical signs

(2) Demonstration of the predisposing cause

d) Treatment

(1) Correct the predisposing factor(s).

(2) If no ulceration is present, give antibiotic/steroid ointments QID initially.

e) Prognosis—depends on the predisposing factors

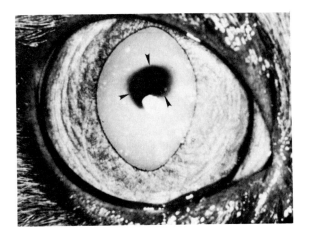

Fig.   8-10. Eighteen-month-old DSH female with unilateral corneal sequestrum (arrows).

3. Corneal sequestration of cats (corneal sequestrum, corneal nigrum, corneal mummification, focal degeneration)—may be ulcerated (Fig. 8-10)
    a) Etiology—essentially unknown
        (1) Chronic irritation
        (2) Prominent eye may predispose
        (3) Most probable cause—dark pigment produced by polymerization of oxidation products of:
            i) Tyrosine
            ii) Dopa
            iii) Epinephrine
            iv) Catechol
            v) Others
        (4) Similar lesions have been described in humans as a result of prolonged use of topical epinephrine.
    b) Clinical signs
        (1) Black, hard, variable-depth plaques, axial or paraaxial
        (2) Epiphora
        (3) Blepharospasms
        (4) Chemosis—variable
        (5) Corneal vascularization
            i) Deep
            ii) Superficial
        (6) Little or no photophobia
        (7) Unresponsive to medical therapy
    c) Diagnosis
        (1) By observation
        (2) Biopsy—excisional, if possible
    d) Treatment

        (1) Keratectomy
            i) Superficial if shallow
            ii) Care must be taken to prevent perforation if the lesion
               is deep
        (2) Treat as a fresh ulceration after operation (see p. 158—Superficial ulceration)
    e) Prognosis
        (1) Superficial lesions—excellent to good
        (2) Deep lesions—poor to guarded
  4. Eosinophilic keratitis of cats
    a) Etiology—unknown, but considered a part of the eosinophilic granuloma complex
    b) Clinical signs
        (1) Proliferative granuloma-like lesion adjacent to the limbus
        (2) Usually bilateral but can be unilateral
        (3) Incidious but continual growth that will progress to blindness
        (4) Usually painless
        (5) When severe, exudate accumulates in the interpalpebral space
    c) Diagnosis
        (1) Clinical signs
        (2) Biopsy—necessary before treating
            i) Eosinophils—pathognomonic
            ii) Lymphocytes, plasma cells—highly suggestive
            iii) Histiocytes and PMNs often seen with above cells
    d) Treatment
        (1) Topical antibiotic/steroid preparation used with moderate success
        (2) Megestrol acetate at decreasing dosage—very effective without adverse effects
            i) 0.5 mg/kg/day for 3 days
            ii) 0.25 mg/kg/day for 3 days
            iii) 0.25 mg/kg q48h for three treatments
            iv) 0.25 mg/kg q72h for three treatments
             v) Continue to decrease until lesions are under control.
            vi) Rarely can therapy be discontinued completely.
    e) Prognosis—excellent
  5. Epithelial inclusion cysts and/or abscess formation—rare
    a) Etiology—previous trauma or ulceration
    b) Clinical signs
        (1) Elevation on cornea—variable size
        (2) Intact cornea
        (3) Opacity values in color; may appear yellow, red, or whitish
        (4) Usually no subjective signs of pain
    c) Diagnosis

          (1) Clinical signs

          (2) Histopathologic diagnosis

        d) Treatment

          (1) Superficial keratectomy

          (2) Treat as an uncomplicated superficial ulceration after surgery

        e) Prognosis—excellent

      6. Interstitial keratitis

        a) Etiologies—secondary lesions

          (1) Infectious canine hepatitis

            i) Natural infection

            ii) Immunization against CAV I

          (2) Ocular wounds or surgery

          (3) Extension of superficial keratitis

          (4) Focal infection of the teeth, prostate, sinuses, kidney, ears, etc.

          (5) Extension of scleritis or neoplasia

          (6) Mycosis

        b) Clinical signs

          (1) Corneal opacity

            i) Does not clear with hypertonic solutions

            ii) Due to edema and cellular infiltration

            iii) Ground glass appearance

            iv) Usually diffuse but can be local

          (2) Vascularization

            i) Circumlimbal ciliary injection

            ii) Superficial vascularization may be present if the lesion is an extension of corneal or scleral disease.

          (3) Pain—varies, depending on the cause

            i) Acute attacks may be extremely painful.

            ii) Postvaccinal attacks may be painless.

          (4) Blindness if opacity and/or anterior uveitis is severe

          (5) May predispose to glaucoma, especially in sight hounds

        c) Diagnosis

          (1) Clinical signs

          (2) Laboratory work-up appropriate for the lesions observed

        d) Treatment

          (1) Directed toward primary cause

          (2) Treat anterior uveitis (see p. 197 Uveitis)

          (3) Treat for secondary glaucoma (see p. 215 Glaucoma)

        e) Prognosis—varies, depending on the primary disease

IV. Dystrophy and degeneration (see Table 4-1)

  A. Epithelial and stromal dystrophy (lipidosis)—familial, bilateral, often symmetric, noninflammatory corneal opacities (Fig. 8-11)

    1. Etiology—presumed hereditary, mode unknown

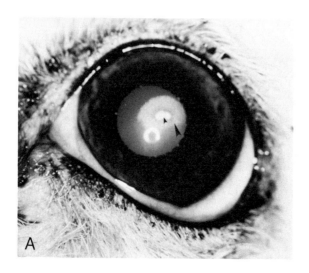

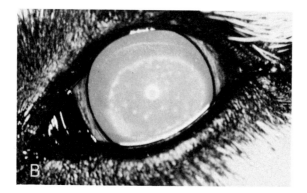

Fig. 8-11. (A) Six-year-old male poodle with superficial corneal dystrophy bilateral. Small arrow identifies dense center; large arrow identifies less dense outer ring. This simulates a bulls eye. (B) Ten-month-old male Siberian husky with bilateral superficial corneal dystrophy. (C) Two-year-old DSH female with bilateral superficial corneal dystrophy, cause unknown.

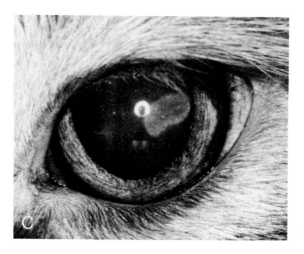

2. Breed predisposition (see Figs. 8-11 A&B, Table 4-1 and Suggested Readings)
3. Clinical signs
   a) Bilateral lesions have a ground glass appearance and may be:
      (1) Static
      (2) Progressive
      (3) Regressive (rarely)
   b) May be opalescent
   c) Central or paracentral
   d) Diffuse or focal
   e) Ring-shaped, racetrack, or other design
   f) Painless
   g) Little or no impairment of sight
4. Diagnosis
   a) Clinical signs
   b) Signalment and history
5. Treatment
   a) None if vision is not compromised
   b) Superficial keratectomy if vision is significantly impaired and lesion is superficial
   c) Penetrating keratoplasty—difficult and expensive
   d) No medical therapy is effective
6. Prognosis
   a) For vision—good
   b) The animal should not be used for breeding
B. Endothelial dystrophy (see Table 4-1)
   1. Etiology—inherited—method unknown
   2. Breed and age predelection—usually occurs in animals 5 years of age or older
      a) Boston terrier (Fig. 8-12)
      b) Chihuahua
      b) Wire-haired terrier
      c) Airedale—observed one dog in my practice
      d) Dachshund
   3. Clinical signs
      a) Usually starts in the dorsal temporal aspects
      b) Most frequently bilateral but can be unilateral
      c) Early—painless
      d) Opaque cornea is thickened due to edema
      e) Lesions progress
         (1) The entire cornea becomes opaque.
         (2) The small vesicles appear superficially.
         (3) The vesicles coalesce to form large bullae.
         (4) The bullae rupture, resulting in painful ulceration.
         (5) Keratoconus results.

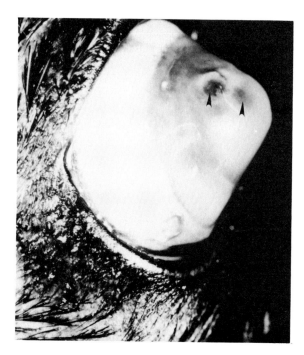

Fig. 8-12. Eight-year-old male Boston terrier with bilateral keratoconus due to endothelial dystrophy. Arrows identify "thinned" corneal regions due to recurrent rupture of vesicles.

        (6) Rupture and blindness are irreparable.

        (7) The lesions will progress to phthisis bulbi.

    4. Diagnosis—by observation, signalment, and history

    5. Treatment

       a) Topical hyperosmotic agents

          (1) Slows progression

          (2) Does not cure the disease

          (3) Dehydrates corneal stroma by osmotic gradients

          (4) 5% NaCl ophthalmic ointment q12h to q4h

       b) Surgery

          (1) Corneal transplant—unsuccessful in my practice

          (2) Conjunctival flap

             i) Alternative method of dehydrating cornea

             ii) Causes opaque cornea but saves the eye

    6. Prognosis—generally poor

       a) Lesions identified and treated early have a better but poor prognosis.

       b) Late—grave

  C. Degenerations

    1. Lipid corneal degeneration (Fig. 8-13)

       a) Etiologies—essentially unknown

          (1) Considered secondary to some corneal injury or insult

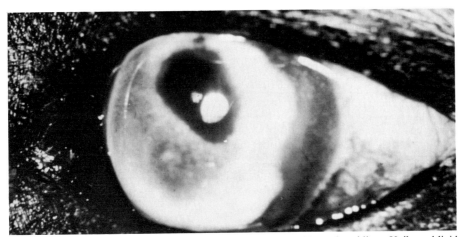

Fig. 8-13. Six-year-old female German shepherd with confirmed hypothyroidism. Unilateral lipid degeneration.

          (2) May be due to metabolic errors in fat metabolism
- b) Clinical signs
  - (1) Usually unilateral
  - (2) A vascular response is manifest.
  - (3) Lesions are elevated above the surrounding cornea.
  - (4) Opacities are dense and appear soap-like.
  - (5) Usually painless
  - (6) May impair vision
- c) Diagnosis
  - (1) Clinical signs
  - (2) Identification of previous corneal injury
  - (3) Identification of systemic lipid metabolic error
- d) Treatment
  - (1) Identify and treat systemic disease.
    - i) Corneal lesions are not reversible when the systemic disease is controlled.
    - ii) Prevents progression
  - (2) Superficial keratectomy is indicated when vision is impaired.
  - (3) Treat as an uncomplicated ulcer after surgery.
  - (4) Topical steroids are indicated when epithelialization occurs.
- e) Prognosis
  - (1) Depends on the predisposing disease
  - (2) The corneal lesion has a good prognosis.
2. Calcium degeneration
  - a) Etiologies
    - (1) Associated with previous corneal injury as in lipid degeneration

    (2) Secondary to parotid duct transposition
    (3) Alteration of pH
    (4) Systemic hypercalcemia (?)
    (5) Hypervitaminosis (?)
    (6) Uremia (?)
  b) Clinical signs
    (1) Extremely dense corneal elevations
    (2) Vascular (inflammatory) components
    (3) Small deposits coalescing to form nodules on surface of cornea (parotid duct transplantation)
    (4) Usually uncomfortable or overtly painful
    (5) Pannus formation as a result of irritation
  c) Diagnosis
    (1) Clinical signs
    (2) Biopsy and identification of:
      i) Calcium carbonate
      ii) Calcium phosphate
  d) Treatment
    (1) Eliminate the cause.
    (2) Apply chelate calcium salts with EDTA.
      i) 10 drops of EDTA in 15 ml of Adapt (Alcon/B.P.) q4h to q6h
      ii) Deeper lesions—superficial epithelial abrasion—0.1-mol/L solution of EDTA applied to cornea for 10 minutes, then scraped off or irrigated to remove salt
    (3) Treat as an ulcer, with broad-spectrum antibiotic ointment.
    (4) After epithelialization, steroids may be used.
  e) Prognosis—depends on cause, but usually guarded
3. Superficial punctate keratitis (Fig. 8-14)
  a) Etiology—unknown (placed here because of the inflammatory component)
  b) Breed predisposition
    (1) Shetland sheepdog—most common in my practice
    (2) Dachshund
    (3) Poodles
  c) Clinical signs
    (1) Multifocal punctate superficial white opacities
    (2) Corneal "facets," which tend to hold fluorescein in absence of ulceration
    (3) Most frequently bilateral but can be unilateral
    (4) Mild conjunctival injection
    (5) Slight epiphora
    (6) Superficial corneal vascularization
    (7) In general, few irritative signs
  d) Diagnosis

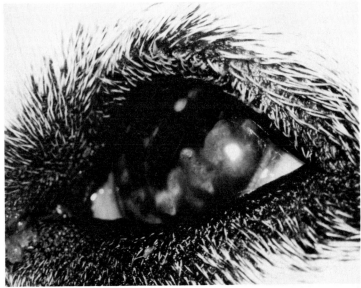

Fig. 8-14. Four-year-old female Shetland sheepdog with bilateral superficial punctate keratitis responsive to topical steroids.

        (1) Clinical signs
        (2) History and signalment
     e) Treatment
        (1) Topical steroids—include antibiotics
           i) Start at q4h to q6h.
           ii) Decrease at weekly intervals until control level is achieved.
           iii) Treat periodically—complete remission is rare in my experience.
     f) Prognosis—good for control
 V. Corneal trauma
   A. Lacerations—most common
     1. Etiologies
       a) Bite wounds
       b) Cuts and scratches
       c) Projectiles (e.g., gunshot)
       d) Direct blows
     2. Clinical signs
       a) Corneal defects visible
       b) Hemorrhage in anterior chamber
       c) Serosanguineus exudate
       d) Pain
          (1) Blepharospasm

        (2) Epiphora

        (3) Change in attitude

     e) Prolapsed uvea

     f) Chemosis

3. Diagnosis—by observation

4. Treatment

     a) Requires surgical repair

        (1) Reappose the lacerated margins.

        (2) Prolapsed uvea

           i) Acute injuries—replace uvea

           ii) Chronic injuries—amputate the prolapsed uvea

        (3) Irrigate the anterior chamber with warmed BSS (Alcon).

        (4) Place simple interrupted sutures intrastromally.

           i) Start from both ends and work toward the center.

           ii) Do not close until several sutures are placed.

           iii) Use 6-0 or 7-0 chromic gut.

        (5) Close the defect and reform the anterior chamber with warmed BSS and a small bubble of air.

        (6) If lesion extends to the limbus:

           i) Perform fornix-based conjunctival flap procedure.

           ii) Examine the limbal area to determine whether the laceration extends to and through the limbus into the sclera.

     b) After operation, treat the lesion as an anterior uveitis.

5. Prognosis

     a) Cats—in general, better prognosis than dogs

     b) Depends on the extent of damage

        (1) Minimal—excellent for sight and cosmesis

        (2) Extensive—guarded for sight and cosmesis

VI. Corneal neoplasms—primary—rare

   A. Fibrous histiocytoma (nodular episcleritis, diffuse episcleritis, nodular fasciitis, inflammatory granuloma, conjunctival granuloma, third eyelid granuloma, and proliferative keratoconjunctivitis)—truly a lesion of the sclera; spreads by extension (see Suggested Readings)

     1. Breed predisposition

        a) Collie—most common breed in my practice (Fig. 8-15)

        b) Border collie

        c) Dalmation

        d) Others, including mixed breeds

     2. Clinical signs

        a) Pink, fleshy mass extending into the cornea from the sclera—may be pigmented

        b) Bilateral or unilateral

        c) May involve the membrana nictitans

        d) May involve the lids

        e) Usually arises from the sclera or episclera

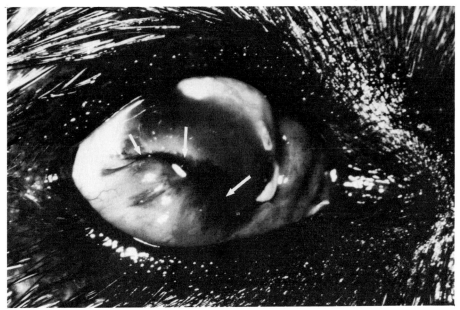

Fig. 8-15. Five-year-old male collie with bilateral fibrous histiocytoma confirmed by biopsy. Arrows outline primary mass.

       f) Usually painless
       g) Some degree of exudate, but not common
       h) May be deforming or blinding in advanced conditions
       i) May have an associated degenerative lipidosis
    3. Diagnosis
       a) By observation and clinical signs
       b) Biopsy—histiocytes, fibrocytes, plasma cells, and lymphocytes
    4. Treatment
       a) Surgical excision
       b) Azathioprine 2 mg/kg/day (see Suggested Readings)
       c) Ancillary therapy—antibiotic/steroid topically applied q6h to q8h
    5. Prognosis
       a) Medical therapy—good—azathioprine may have to be continued and blood parameters monitored for drug toxicity
       b) Surgery—poor results in my practice—required for confirmation of the disease
  B. Viral papillomatosis (Fig. 5-13)
    1. Etiology—virus
    2. Clinical signs
       a) Elevated, rough, pinkish or whitish mass
       b) Secondary lesions due to irritation

   c) The lesions are variable in size
   d) Occurs in young dogs
   3. Diagnosis
      a) Clinical signs
      b) Biopsy
   4. Treatment
      a) Surgical excision
      b) Immunization with commercially available vaccine
      c) Some are self-limiting
   5. Prognosis—excellent
C. Other neoplasms
   1. Classification—may be primary or secondary
      a) Malignant melanoma—invades by extension
      b) Squamous cell carcinoma—more common in cats
      c) Hemangiosarcoma
      d) Fibrosarcoma
      e) Lymphoma
      f) Basal cell carcinoma
   2. Clinical signs
      a) All are similar, with elevations and corneal distortion
      b) Pigment and vascular or inflammatory response varies
      c) Pain—none to severe
   3. Diagnosis
      a) Clinical signs
      b) Biopsy
   4. Treatment
      a) Surgical extirpation
      b) Enucleation or evisceration may be indicated
   5. Prognosis—depends on the neoplasm

DISEASES OF THE SCLERA

I. Congenital—staphyloma—a protrusion of the fibrous tunic lined with uvea
   (Fig. 8-16 and Fig. 8-17).
   A. Clinical signs
      1. Observed most often in collies (see p. 241—Collie eye anomaly)
      2. Can be seen with an ophthalmoscope
      3. Due to:
         a) Incomplete closure of the embryonic fissure
         b) Lack of development of mesodermal coats of the eye (i.e., collie
            eye anomaly)
   B. Predisposed breeds
      1. Collies
      2. Shetland sheepdog

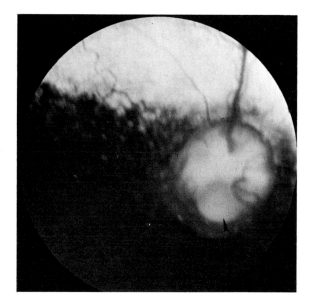

Fig. 8-16. White male German shepherd puppy with a coloboma of the optic disc (arrow).

      3. Basenji
      4. German shepherd (Fig. 8-16)
      5. Australian shepherd
      6. Rarely in cats
   C. Diagnosis—made by observation
   D. Treatment—none
   E. Prognosis—good for sight but probably inherited, so affected animals should not be used in any breeding program
II. Inflammatory lesions

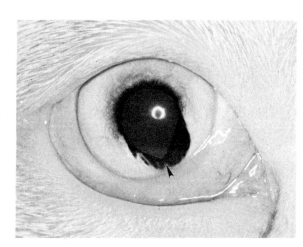

Fig. 8-17. Great Dane puppy with multiple ocular anomalies, including an iris coloboma (arrow).

A. General
  1. Isolated lesions are rare and difficult to identify
  2. Usually there are other tissues involved
     a) Conjunctiva
     b) Cornea
     c) Uvea
     d) Retina
     e) Episclera and extrinsic muscles
B. Diseases
  1. Many diseases have minor clinical differences but similar histologic characteristics
     a) Preferred term—fibrous histiocytoma
     b) Synonyms
        (1) Nodular episcleritis
        (2) Diffuse episcleritis
        (3) Nodular episcleritis
        (4) Inflammatory granuloma
        (5) Necrogranulomatous sclerouveitis
  2. Clinical signs
     a) Focal or diffuse scleritis or episcleritis
     b) Fibrovascular elevations may extend onto the cornea.
     c) The third eyelid may be involved.
     d) Often bilateral but can be unilateral
     e) Pain is minimal unless the lesion is advanced.
  3. Diagnosis
     a) Clinical signs
     b) Biopsy—fibroblasts, histiocytes, lymphoctes, and plasma cells
  4. Treatment
     a) Surgical biopsy to confirm diagnosis
     b) Azathioprine 2 mg/kg/day
        (1) Monitor the CBC for evidence of bone marrow depression.
        (2) Monitor serum chemistries for elevated liver enzymes.
     c) Topical antibiotic/steroid ointment may be used as adjunctive therapy.
  5. Prognosis
     a) Usually good to excellent
     b) Severe lesions—guarded
C. Trauma—usually results in tears (Fig. 8-18)
  1. Clinical signs
     a) Overt signs of penetrating injury
        (1) Hyphema
        (2) Uveal prolapse
        (3) Vitreal hemorrhage
        (4) Soft, deformed globe
     b) May result in traumatic staphyloma

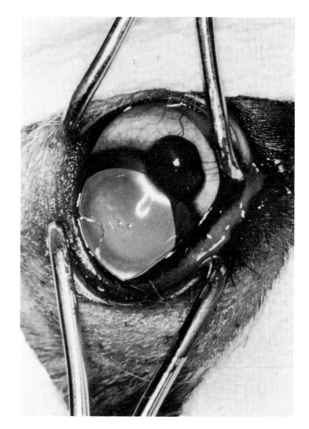

Fig. 8-18. Three-year-old terrier-type male with a traumatic injury resulting in an iris and ciliary body prolapse; patient prepared for surgical repair.

2. Diagnosis—by observation
3. Treatment—for simple injury
   a) Surgical closure
   b) Control inflammation with:
      (1) Antiprostaglandin
      (2) Corticosteroid
   c) Systemic antibiotics
4. Prognosis
   a) Severe—guarded
   b) Uncomplicated simple injury (rare)—good

SUGGESTED READINGS

Bistner SI, Aguirre G, Shively JN: Hereditary corneal dystrophy in the Manx cat. Proc ACVO 5:87, 1974

Roberts SR, Bistner SI: Persistent pupillary membranes in Basenji dogs. J Am Vet Med Assoc 153:523, 1968

Severin GA: Veterinary Ophthalmology Notes. 2nd Ed. Colorado State University Press, Fort Collins, 1976

Smith J, Bistner S, Riis R: Infiltrative corneal lesions resembling fibrous histiocytoma: clinical and pathologic findings in six dogs and one cat. J Am Vet Med Assoc 169:722, 1976

9

Uvea

ANATOMY AND PHYSIOLOGY

The uvea is the pigmented vascular tunic located between the fibrous and nervous tunics. It has three major components: the iris, the ciliary body, and the choroid.

Iris

The iris is a diaphragm separating the anterior and posterior chambers. The dog's central aperature (pupil) is round. The cat's is slit-like in a vertical direction when constricted, but round when dilated. The iris varies in thickness, being thinnest at its base and thickest near the collarette. The pupillary margin rests on a "cushion" of aqueous overlying the lens. The pupillary margin is slightly anterior to the remaining anterior surface of the iris. When the lens is absent or displaced posteriorly, the posterior displacement of the iris results in a deep anterior chamber. The iris trembles (iridodenesis) with the slightest eye movement as a result of the lack of lens support.

Iris color varies, ranging from dark brown, particularly common in dogs, to light blue. The predominant color in cats is golden yellow or green. The color is determined by the concentration of stromal pigment and the cellular arrangement of the anterior surface (anterior border layer) of the iris. The anterior border layer (the endothelium) is composed of tightly or loosely arranged stromal cells. The tighter arrangement provides a smoother, darker surface than the loose arrangement observed in a light-colored iris.

The stroma consists of pigmented and nonpigmented cells, collagen fibrils, blood vessels, nerves, and a matrix of mucopolysaccharides.

The sphincter and dilator muscles have all the characteristics of smooth muscle but are neuroectodermal in origin. They are believed to have migrated from the neuroepithelium of the developing optic cup. Sphincter muscle fiber arrangement differs little in all species, but these differences result in variations of pupil shape. The cat's sphincter muscle fibers are interwoven vertically in the dorsal and ventral regions, resulting in the slit-like appearance when constricted. The dog's, on the other hand, are concentrically arranged, resulting in a round pupil when constricted. The sphincter is innervated by parasympathetic nerve fibers.

The dilator muscle extends radially from the iris base to the pupil, separating the stroma from the pigmented epithelial layers. The muscle is said to be derived from the anterior layer of the pigment epithelium and may contain melanin granules. Sympathetic nerve fibers innervate the dilator, and contraction results in a large pupil (mydriasis).

The pigmented epithelium is derived from the anterior portion of the embryonic optic cup and has a double layer, part of which is modified to smooth muscle (see page 187). The pupillary margin is lined by this heavily pigmented tissue seen on gross examination as the pupillary ruff. The anterior layer continues over the ciliary body as the pigmented layer and ultimately as the retinal pigment epithelium. The posterior layer is continuous with the nonpigmented ciliary epithelium and the neuroepithelium posteriorly.

The long posterior ciliary arteries terminate as the temporal and nasal arteries of the iris and join one another at the 12 o'clock and 6 o'clock positions, forming the basilar iridal artery. This artery can be seen in the normal dog's and cat's eye.

Ciliary Body

The ciliary body forms an asymmetric girdle, wider in the temporal and ventral regions than in the nasal and dorsal aspects. On gross examination it appears triangular, with the outer surface adjacent to the sclera, the inner surface adjacent to the vitreous and lens, and the base adjacent to the origin of the iris, iridocorneal angle, and uveal trabecular meshwork (Fig. 9-1). The apex, or posterior border of the ciliary body, continues posteriorly as the choroid.

The ciliary body can be divided into the pars plicata (ciliary processes) and the pars plana. The ciliary processes are fin-like structures covered by two layers of neuroepithelium. The layer adjacent to the vitreous is nonpigmented and continues posteriorly as the neural retina, while the layer closest to the

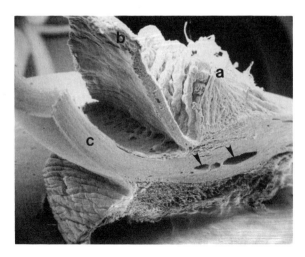

Fig. 9-1. Scanning electron micrograph of ciliary body and associated structures. (×20) a, ciliary processes; b, iris; c, cornea. Arrows indicate intrascleral plexus.

vascular core is pigmented and continues as the retinal pigmented epithelium. The apices of the pigmented and nonpigmented epithelial cells are joined by tight junctions; these contribute to the blood aqueous barrier. The two layers are thrown into folds that are deeper anteriorly and shallower posteriorly, giving a triangular appearance to the ciliary body (see Fig. 9-1). Within these folds are vessels that are continuous with those of the choriocapillaris and separated from the pigment epithelium by a basement membrane and collagen fibrils. The vessels and the arrangement of the two layers of epithelial cells and their enzyme systems form the secretory structure for aqueous production.

The pars plana is the flat, thin, posterior portion of the ciliary body. The surface adjacent to the vitreous has two layers of epithelium, as the ciliary processes described above, and they too possess tight junctions at their apices. Within the pars plana are muscles of accommodation. Posteriorly they are thin, but they become thicker and more prominent anteriorly, toward the base of the ciliary body. The predominant muscle in carnivores is the longitudinal muscle. In primates, the circular and oblique muscles are also well developed. The lack of development of these muscles in carnivores results in a much smaller structure than that in primates. The ciliary muscle arrangement splits the ciliary body into two leaves: the outer leaf, the cribiform ligament, hugs the sclera and extends anteriorly to Descemet's membrane; the inner leaf runs forward toward the root of the iris. The two leaves form a cleft, the ciliary cleft, or cilioscleral sinus. The canal of Schlemm, found in primates, could be considered an analogous structure. The ciliary cleft contains fine fibers referred to as the ciliary trabecular meshwork. These are insertional fibers of the longitudinal muscles of the ciliary body.

Choroid

The choroid (posterior uvea) is composed of, from the outermost layer in: the lamina fusca (suprachoroidea); the large choroidal vessel layer; the tapetum (cellular in carnivores); and the choriocapillaris.

The choroid provides nourishment to the outer retinal layers. The stroma is heavily pigmented and provides the "heat sink" effect of the eyeground. The pigment, which is dark brown, is found in the interstices of the choroidal vasculature. This, in addition to the pigmented epithelium of the retina, provides the dark brown or black color of the fundus, except in the area of the tapetum.

The carnivore tapetum is a cellular structure 1 to 12 or 15 cells thick. It is roughly triangular in outline, often approximating a right scalene triangle, in the dog and is rounded in the cat. The tapetum occupies the dorsal half of the fundus and constitutes about one-third of the eyeground. Tapetal size varies by breed and species. Toy breeds of dogs have smaller tapeta than sight hounds, working dogs, or cats. Some animals may be atapetal as an atypical variant of normal. There is no definitive pigment in the cellular tapetum, and the color observed is due to specific spectral absorption and reflection. Most of the light entering the eye and projected to the tapetum penetrates its surface and is scattered within its cellular matrix. Some is absorbed selectively, and the remainder emerges from the surface. This reflected light determines the tapetal color observed with the ophthalmoscope. Analogous to this phenomenon is the prism effect of white light entering the prism and separating the colors into their respective wave lengths on exiting it. The color of the tapetal-reflected light varies by species, animals, age, thickness of the tapetal cells. This can be appreciated by observing, for example, the green margin and yellow-green center of the tapetum commonly observed in a dog's eye. The tapetum is thinner peripherally than centrally, and the spectral absorption–reflection phenomenon differs due to the concentration of the cells. The internal limiting membrane of the retina give the tapetum a "polished" surface. The concavity functions as a parabolic reflector, resulting in a brilliant reflection. The function of the tapetum teleologically is to conserve light. I believe the tapetum functions as a macular potentiator by reflecting the most receptor-sensitive light rays back to the rods and cones and enhancing the predators vision in the superior fundus or ventral visual field.

DISEASES OF THE UVEA

Anterior Uvea (Iris and Ciliary Body)

I. Inherited or congenital
   A. Persistent pupillary membrane (PPM) (see Table 4-1)
      1. Etiology
         a) Inherited
            (1) Basenjis (Fig. 9-2A)
               i) Mode of inheritance is unknown
               ii) My experimental breeding trials were inconclusive because of the unknown status of the foundation animals.
                   (A) Foundation animals may have been affected as puppies and appeared normal as adults.
                   (B) Investigators must start with a foundation colony of affected puppies and evaluate specific ratios of affected animals produced by them.
                   (C) Animals must be outcrossed to another breed in which the condition has never been identified.
            (2) May also be inherited in other dogs, but there is no conclusive evidence
            (3) No evidence exists to support inheritance in cats
         b) Congenital
            (1) Occurs in many species (Fig. 9-2B)
            (2) Cause is unknown

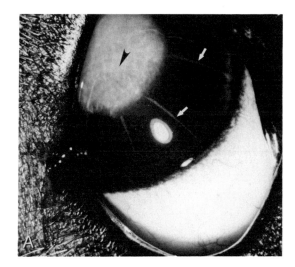

Fig. 9-2. (A) Basenji puppy with persistent pupillary strands (membrane) and secondary corneal opacity (black arrow) and strands (white arrows). (B) Two-year-old DSH female with bilateral persistent pupillary strands (membranes). Notice where they arise from the surface of the iris; compare with Figure 9-12.

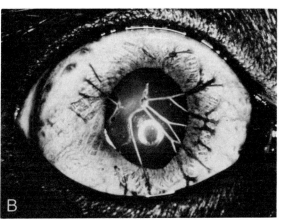

2. Clinical signs
   a) Remnants of the pupillary membrane are visible—they radiate from the collarette (see Fig. 9-2B) to:
      (1) Lens—may predispose to cataracts
      (2) Bridge the pupil and attach to opposite collarette
      (3) Insert onto the corneal endothelium—results in corneal opacity of variable degree (see Fig. 9-2A)
   b) Presence of a small central cluster of stellate pigment cells on the anterior lens capsule
      (1) Seen often in miniature schnauzers, poodles, cocker spaniels, and others
      (2) Nonprogressive
      (3) Does not interfere with vision

           (4) Must be differentiated from postinflammatory pigmented rests
      c) Often associated with other ocular anomalies in basenjis
      d) All kittens and puppies have remnants of the pupillary membrane at birth and when their eyes open.
           (1) They continue to atrophy with maturation.
           (2) When not adherent to other structures, they are not pathologic.
   3. Diagnosis—made by observation
   4. Treatment—none
   5. Prognosis (sight)
      a) If secondary cataracts or corneal opacities do not exist—excellent
      b) If cataracts or blinding corneal opacities exist—grave (see Fig. 9-2A)
      c) Affected animals, particularly basenjis, should not be used as breeding animals
B. Colobomas
   1. Etiology—unknown, but may be associated with other multiple ocular anomalies of an inherited nature (see Fig. 8-16)
   2. Clinical signs
      a) Typical
           (1) Notch-like defect in the inferonasal iris (see Fig. 8-17)
           (2) Pupil irregular due to defect, including pupillary margin
           (3) Full-thickness
               i) No visible iridal tissue in the defect
               ii) May have an associated ciliary coloboma and absence of lenticular zonules
           (4) Partial-thickness
               i) Brown irides—defect appears lighter-colored (i.e., tan)
               ii) Light-colored irides—defect appears black or gray
           (5) May appear as a misplaced pupil (corectopia) (see Fig. 8-17)
      b) Atypical
           (1) Similar characteristics to those of typical colobomas but occur anywhere in the iris
           (2) Pseudopolycoria
               i) Multiple holes
                   (*A*) Complete or incomplete
                   (*B*) Unilateral or bilateral
               ii) No definite sphincter muscle around false pupil
               iii) Appearance alters as true pupillary size changes
               iv) No clinical manifestation of visual dysfunction
               v) Must be differentiated from iris atrophy (Fig. 1-3)

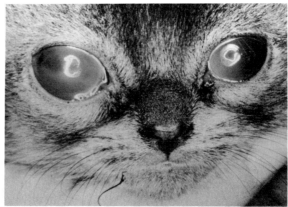

Fig. 9-3. Persian kitten (one of a litter of four, all affected). All had associated glaucoma in one or both eyes. Presumed due to lack of angle development and absence of iris (aniridia).

      (*A*) Colobomas seen in young animals

      (*B*) Atrophy develops after inflammatory disease or primary essential atrophy with age

   c) Often associated with multiple-ocular anomalies (Fig. 8-17)

      (1) Microphthalmia

      (2) Color dilution defects (i.e., Waardenburg's syndrome in cats)

  2. Diagnosis—by observation

  3. Treatment—none—animal should not be used for breeding

  4. Prognosis

    a) Uncomplicated lesions—excellent

    b) Multiple ocular anomalies—poor

C. Aniridia—extremely rare—I have observed it in only one litter of Persian kittens (Fig. 9-3)

  1. Etiology—unknown, usually associated with multiple ocular anomalies

  2. Clinical signs

    a) No visible iris—histologically, there may be hyoplastic or dysplastic iridal tissue

    b) Often associated with an increase in intraocular pressure

      (1) Defect in angle development

      (2) Defect in corneal development

    c) Blind in eyes with glaucoma

    d) May be unilateral or bilateral

  3. Diagnosis—by observation

  4. Treatment—none

  5. Prognosis—grave

D. Heterochromia irides

  1. Nomenclature—I use the term to describe bicolored irides (one or both)

    2. Etiology
       a) May be associated with the merling gene
         (1) Collie
         (2) Shetland sheepdog
         (3) Australian shepherd
         (4) Harlequin Great Dane (see Fig. 8-17)
         (5) Others
       b) Incomplete development or absence of pigment in the iridal stroma
    3. Clinical signs
       a) A blue or light color segment in an otherwise brown iris
       b) One iris blue, the other brown
       c) No visual dysfunction is manifest
       d) Pupillary response is normal
    4. Diagnosis—by observation
    5. Treatment—none
    6. Prognosis—excellent
E. Predominately white coat, blue eyes, and deafness in dogs and cats (Waardenburg's syndrome in humans)
    1. Etiology
       a) Cats—dominant, with complete penetrance for white fur, incomplete penetrance for blue irides and deafness
       b) Dogs—There is no conclusive evidence for the method of inheritance, but it may be associated with the inheritability of coat color.
    2. Clinical signs
       a) Cats
         (1) Predominately white fur
         (2) One or both irides are blue
         (3) Lack of choroidal pigmentation in one or both eyes
         (4) Atapetal—unilateral or bilateral
         (5) Deafness
         (6) Possible decreased or impaired night vision
         (7) Possible decreased fertility
       b) Dogs
         (1) Usually multiple ocular anomalies (see Figs. 8-17 and 11-5)
           i) Iridodysgenesis
             (*A*) Decreased stromal pigmentation
             (*B*) Large anomalous iridal vessels
             (*C*) Hypoplastic or anomalous sphincter and dilator muscles
             (*D*) Iris hypoplasia
           ii) Goniodysgenesis
             (*A*) Thickened iridal base

              (*B*) Mesodermal bands spanning the angle
              (*C*) Includes ciliary body and drainage channels
        iii) Hypoplasia of the trabecular meshwork and absence of the cilioscleral sinus
        iv) Hypoplasia of ciliary body and musculature
         v) Hypopigmentation of ciliary epithelium
        vi) Variable degrees of retinal dysplasia
       vii) Microphthalmia bilateral or unilateral
      viii) Staphylomas—variable
        ix) Hypoplasia of ganglion cell layer with resulting optic nerve hypoplasia
    (2) Partial albinism
    (3) Deafness
  3. Diagnosis—by observation
  4. Treatment—none—owners should be advised against repeat matings
  5. Prognosis
    a) Cats—excellent to good
    b) Dogs—poor to grave
F. Partial or complete albinism and multiple ocular anomalies without deafness
  1. Etiology—inherited, but mode unknown
    a) May be a less expressive manifestation of that associated with deafness
    b) White and merle traits are autosomal dominant
    c) Ocular lesions not always present in white or merle animals
      (1) More research is necessary to identify completely etiopathogenesis of this phenomenon
      (2) Albinism in humans
         i) Inherited
        ii) Normal amounts of melanin are not produced
           (*A*) Metabolic disorder
           (*B*) Tyrosine is not converted to 3,4-dihydroxyphenylalanine
        iii) Albinism, poor vision, nystagmus, but otherwise normal development of the eyes
  2. Clinical signs
    a) Breed predisposition (merling or color dilution factors)
      (1) Collies
      (2) Shetland sheepdogs
      (3) Australian shepherds
      (4) American fox hounds
      (5) Siberian huskies
      (6) Malamutes
      (7) Great Danes

     (8) Dalmatians

     (9) Dachshunds

     (10) Beagles

    b) Similar signs for those with deafness

   3. Diagnosis—by observation

   4. Treatment—none—affected animals or their parents should not be used for breeding

   5. Prognosis—same as for lesions associated with deafness

 G. Absence of pupil (acoria)—rare—reported only in five Saint Bernard puppies

   1. Etiology—unknown, but presumed inherited

   2. Clinical signs—observed in five puppies

    a) Absence of the pupil (acoria)

    b) Microphthalmia—unilateral or bilateral

    c) Buphthalmia (glaucoma)

    d) Anterior synechia

    e) Aphakia (absence of the lens)

    f) Retinal dysplasia

    g) Retinal detachment

    h) Blindness

   3. Diagnosis—by observation

   4. Treatment—none—advise against breeding

   5. Prognosis—grave

 H. Iris cysts (Fig. 9-4)

   1. Etiology

    a) Formed from the neural ectoderm of the rim of the optic cup

    b) Since there is breed predisposition, it may be inherited.

    c) Some may be due to postinflammatory causes

   2. Clinical signs

    a) Predisposed breeds (usually in older animals)

     (1) Basset hounds

     (2) Boston terriers

     (3) Beagles

     (4) Golden retrievers

     (5) English bulldogs

     (6) Brittany spaniels

     (7) Others

    b) Variable-sized spheric bodies in the anterior chamber

     (1) Free-floating

     (2) Attached at the pupillary margin

    c) Transluminate

    d) One or several in one or both eyes

    e) Usually do not cause visual impairment

    f) May rupture and produce a pigmented precipitate on the

     (1) Corneal endothelium—usually ventral

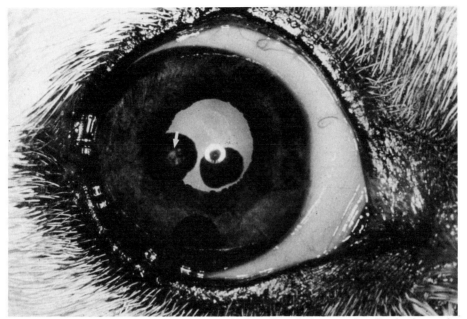

Fig. 9-4. Aged male bassett hound, right eye. Iridal or ciliary body cysts, free-floating in anterior chamber. A cyst (arrow) demonstrates an important differential criterion; it transluminates.

        (2) Anterior lens capsule

   3. Diagnosis—by observation and ability to transluminate sphere

   4. Treatment—none—some people advocate aspiration

      a) Most often contraindicated, in my opinion

      b) Only necessary in the rare instance of visual impairment due to excessive cyst formation

   5. Prognosis—excellent

II. Anterior uveitis (Figs. 9-5, 9-6, and A-2, in Appendix)

  A. Etiologies

    1. Exogenous

      a) Trauma—see Iris prolapse, page 207

        (1) Blunt, nonpenetrating

        (2) Sharp, penetrating

          i) Sticks

          ii) Bite wounds

          iii) Lacerations

            (*A*) Glass

            (*B*) Claws

            (*C*) Other sharp objects

        (3) Surgical or aqueous centesis

      b) Extension from local inflammation

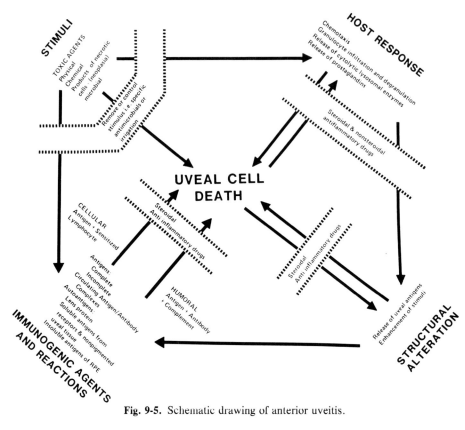

Fig. 9-5. Schematic drawing of anterior uveitis.

    (1) Keratitis
        i) Superficial—caused by an axon reflex
        ii) Deep—caused by release of toxins
    (2) Scleritis
  c) Reaction to foreign bodies in conjunctiva or cornea
  d) Reactions to necrotic neoplasms or byproducts
  e) Reaction to thermal injury to the adnexa
2. Hematogenous (endogenous)
  a) Bacterial disease
    (1) *Brucella canis* (Fig. 9-6)
    (2) Leptospirosis
    (3) *Streptococcus*
    (4) Others
  b) Viral
    (1) Infectious canine hepatitis
    (2) Infectious feline peritonitis
    (3) Feline leukemia virus

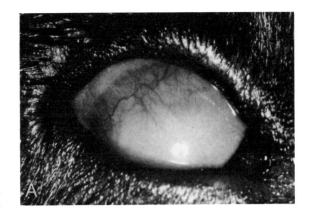

Fig. 9-6. (A) A 21/2-year-old Doberman pinscher spayed female with a severe intraocular inflammatory reaction due to *Brucella canis*, identified by aqueous culture. (B) Gross section through the fixed globe, indicating panuveitis.

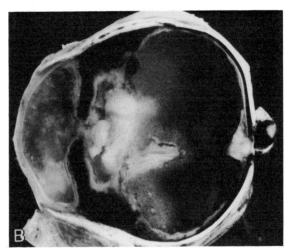

         (4) Distemper
     c) Mycotic
         (1) Histoplasmosis
         (2) Coccidioidomycosis
         (3) Blastomycosis
         (4) Cryptomycosis
         (5) Nocardiosis
         (6) Aspergillosis
         (7) Candidiasis
         (8) Paecilomycosis
     d) Algae—protothecosis
     e) Parasites
         (1) Dirofilariasis
         (2) Rarely, other migrating larvae
     f) Protozoa

    (1) Toxoplasmosis
    (2) Encephalitozoonosis (nosematosis)
  g) Rickettsia
    (1) Ehrlichiosis (tropical canine pancytopenia)
    (2) Leishmaniasis
    (3) *R. rickettsii* (Rocky Mountain spotted fever)
 3. Immune-mediated
  a) Immediate hypersensitivity
    (1) Type I—atopic allergy; acute anaphylaxis
    (2) Type II—cytotoxic hypersensitivity; complement-dependent hypersensitivity
    (3) Type III—Arthus reaction; serum sickness
  b) Delayed hypersensitivity
    (1) Type IV—cell-mediated hypersensitivity
    (2) Type V—stimulatory hypersensitivity
  c) Autoimmunity
    (1) Structural and functional damage produced by the action of immunologically competent cells and antibodies against healthy tissue components
    (2) Often poorly documented in ocular disease
    (3) Examples
     i) Lens-induced uveitis
     ii) Recurrent uveitis
     iii) Vogt–Koyanagi–Harada (VKH) syndrome (Fig. 9-7)
 4. Metabolic diseases—hyperlipoproteinemia—cause or effect?
 5. Idiopathic—a large number of uveitides unfortunately fall into this category
 6. Neoplastic—see Suggested Readings
  a) General
    (1) Early primary neoplasms do not cause severe inflammation, whereas metastatic lesions often are markedly inflammatory.
    (2) Rapidly growing masses result in necrosis, which predisposes to uveal cell death.
  b) Primary neoplasms
    (1) Malignant melanoma (Fig. 9-8)
    (2) Ciliary body adenoma (Fig. 9-9)
    (3) Ciliary body adenocarcinoma
  c) Secondary neoplasms
    (1) Lymphosarcoma (Fig. 9-10)
    (2) Mammary tumors
    (3) Many others
B. Clinical signs—may be acute, chronic, unilateral, or bilateral
 1. Subjective
  a) Epiphora

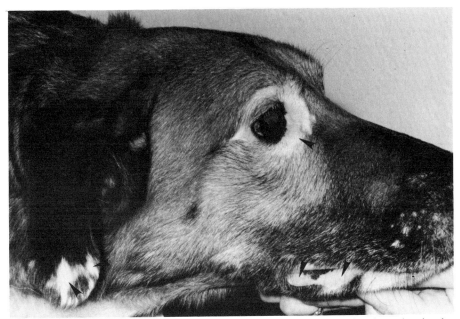

Fig. 9-7. Three-year-old mixed breed male with sequellae to a severe bilateral ocular and periocular inflammatory disease compatible with VKH. Arrows identify vitiligo.

        b) Blepharospasms
        c) Photophobia
        d) Visual deficits—clinically more demonstrable when bilateral
        e) Self-induced trauma
    2. Objective
        a) Corneal opacity—variable
           (1) Edema

Fig. 9-8. Four-year-old golden retriever male with an iridal melanoma, left eye. A sector iridectomy was performed and the histopath was considered benign. A 3-year follow-up indicated no evidence of recurrence.

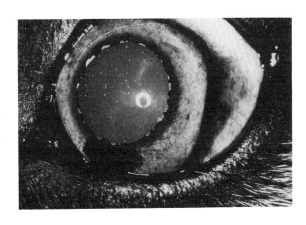

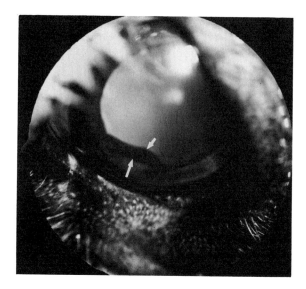

Fig. 9-9. Seven-year-old golden retriever male with a ciliary body adenoma, right eye. Arrows identify enlargement behind the iris. Signs of anterior uveitis were manifest.

(2) Cellular
(3) Keratic precipitates (KPs)
(4) Vascularization
    i) Short, brush-like perilimbal infiltration—"ciliary flush"
    ii) When associated with keratitis, there may be branching (dichotomous) vessels.
b) Conjunctival involvement

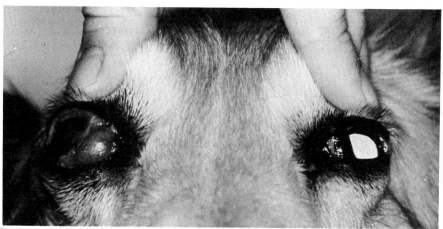

Fig. 9-10. Aged male collie-type dog with bilateral retrobulbar lymphosarcoma. The right eye was more involved.

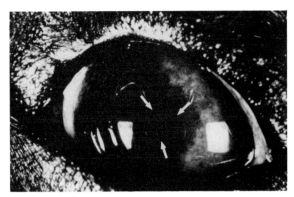

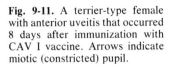

Fig. 9-11. A terrier-type female with anterior uveitis that occurred 8 days after immunization with CAV I vaccine. Arrows indicate miotic (constricted) pupil.

  (1) Chemosis
  (2) Injection
  (3) Inflammation
 c) Enophthalmos
  (1) Due to pain
  (2) Prolapsed third eyelid
  (3) Smaller palpebral fissure (blepharospasm)
 d) Flare—increased specific density of aqueous (plasmoid aqueous) (Figs. 1-1 and 9-11)
 e) Cells in the anterior chamber
  (1) Hyphema—red cells (Fig. 9-12)
  (2) Hypopyon Fig. 8-7—white cells—does not necessarily indicate an intraocular infection
  (3) Fibrin
  (4) Pigment (Fig. 9-13)
 f) Miosis (see Fig. 9-11)
 g) Iris surface
  (1) Swollen
  (2) "Velvety" with loss of crypts and surface morphologic features
  (3) Altered color
    i) Dull
    ii) Red—due to neovascularization (rubeosis irides) or congestion
    iii) Acute—darker
    iv) Chronic—atrophy may result in a thin, almost transparent iris
 h) Abnormal adhesions (synechiae) (Fig. 9-14 and Fig. 9-13)
  (1) Anterior surface of the iris is adherent to cornea
  (2) Posterior surface of the iris is adherent to lens
    i) May result in an irregularly shaped pupil

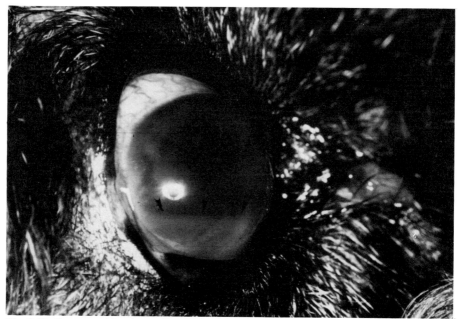

Fig. 9-12. One-year-old male poodle with hyphema (arrows). This area was red due to the RBCs. The cause was unknown.

        ii) Complete annular synechia results in secluding the pupil, ballooning the iris forward (iris bombé) (see Fig. 9-14)

           (*A*) Prevents aqueous from flowing through the pupil from posterior chamber to the anterior chamber

           (*B*) Results in elevated intraocular pressure

     i) Decreased intraocular pressure (hypotony)

        (1) Results from loss of integrity of the ciliary process epithelium

        (2) Must be remembered when recovery occurs, because secondary glaucoma may result when inflammation subsides

     j) Concomitant systemic signs of disease

  C. Diagnosis

    1. Clinical signs

    2. Evidence of systemic disease

      a) History

      b) CBC

      c) Profile

      d) Serology

      e) Immune screen

      f) Radiographs

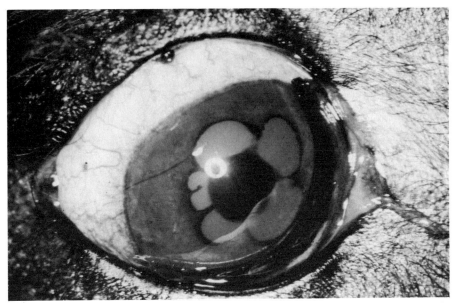

Fig. 9-13. Eight-year-old female poodle with posterior synechiae and pigment deposits on anterior lens capsule, sequellae to anterior uveitis. Compare origin of strands to persistent pupillary membranes in Figure 9-2.

Fig. 9-14. White aged Persian cat with an iris bombé, sequella to anterior uveitis. Arrow identifies anterior bulging of the iris surface. (Courtesy of Dr. Michael T. Doherty, Beavercreek, Oregon.)

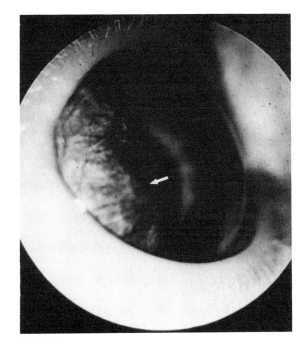

   3. Ultrasonography
   4. Aqueous centesis
      a) Culture
      b) Cytology
      c) Serology
   5. Tonometry
      a) Hypotony—acute (4 to 8 mm Hg)
      b) Normotensive or hypertensive—chronic (>27 mm Hg)
D. Treatment—a specific diagnosis will provide the most effective guide-
   line for treatment
   1. Identify and eliminate causative agent(s).
      a) Treat specifically if agent is known
      b) Often, may not be able to identify
   2. Control inflammatory process.
      a) Topical steroidal antiinflammatory agents
         (1) If the lesion is restricted to the anterior uvea, effective
             levels may be reached with topical administration.
         (2) Dexamethazone—my preference
         (3) Use an ointment base q4h to q6h initially until improved,
             then q6h to q8h
         (4) If solutions are used, double the frequency.
      b) Nonsteroidal antiinflammatory agents (antiprostaglandins)
         (1) Aspirin
             i) 1 grain/10 kg body weight tid for dogs
             ii) 1 grain/10 kg body weight bid for cats
         (2) Banamine (Schering Corp.)—should not be used in cats
             i) IV only
             ii) 0.250 mg/kg once daily
             iii) Do not use with aspirin.
             iv) Do not exceed 5 days.
      c) Atropine SO$_4$ 1%
         (1) Restores the integrity of vascular permeability—mecha-
             nism is unknown
         (2) Prevents complete synechiae
             i) The miotic pupil, "sticky" plasmoid aqueous, and
                cells predispose to annular synechiae.
             ii) When the pupil is dilated, the contact surface area
                 between the iris and lens is decreased.
                 (*A*) This decreases predisposition to pupillary
                      seclusion.
                 (*B*) Miosis may be due to direct effect of prostaglan-
                      dins on smooth muscle, resulting in contraction.
                 (*C*) The pupil should start to dilate before the patient
                      is released to the owner.
             iii) Agents

        (*A*) Mydriatic/cyclopegic—atropine SO$_4$ 1%
           (*1*) Applied to effect
           (*2*) Not an inoccuous drug
              (*a*) Can atropinize an animal
              (*b*) May predispose to decreased lacrimation
           (*3*) Start q4h, then decrease frequency to maintain mydriasis
        (*B*) Mydriatic—phenylephrine 10%—direct acting
        (*C*) Antiprostaglandins—see aspirin and Banamine above
      (3) Eliminate photophobia—mydriatic/cycloplegic—atropine SO$_4$ 1% (see above)
         i) The mydriatic and cycloplegic effects are not equal.
         ii) Decreases the pain associated with spasms of the ciliary muscles
         iii) Phenylephrine is a direct-acting sympathomimetic drug and will *not* cause cycloplegia.

E. Prognosis
    1. Uncomplicated—excellent
    2. Severe systemic disease—guarded
      a) *Brucella canis* (see Fig. 9-6)
      b) Feline infectious peritonitis
      c) Mycosis
    3. Neoplasms—good to grave, depending on type

III. Iris prolapse (Fig. 9-15)
    A. Sequella of penetrating corneal injuries
    B. Iris moves through the defect

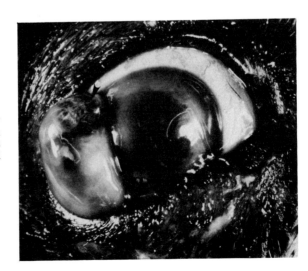

Fig. 9-15. Beagle male puppy trauma inflicted by Siamese cat in the household. Arrow identifies iris surface in bulging damaged cornea.

       1. Plugs the hole
       2. Vascular ischemia
       3. Fibrinous plasmoid aqueous covers surface
  C. Clinical signs
       1. Iris is visible mounded on cornea
         a) Dark color, usually black
         b) Fibrinous, tenacious material covers prolapsed iris
       2. Some corneal edema
         a) Variable
         b) May be clear at the periphery
       3. Anterior chamber may display
         a) Hyphema
         b) Flare
         c) Shallow
         d) Pupil, obscured or eccentric
       4. The prolapsed iris obscures the margin of the wound
         a) If it extends to the limbus, it may include the ciliary body.
         b) Extent must be identified by examining defect under conjunctiva.
  D. Diagnosis—by observation
  E. Treatment
       1. Do not use ointments.
       2. Evaluate for shock and treat appropriately.
       3. Induce general anesthesia.
       4. Irrigate and remove the debris.
       5. Replace the iris with iris repositor, if possible.
       6. Place sutures intrastromally.
         a) Use 6-0 or 7-0 chromic gut.
         b) Place several sutures before tying.
       7. Reform the anterior chamber with Balanced Salt Soltion BSS (Alcon) and a small bubble of air.
       8. Treat as an anterior uveitis.
  F. Prognosis—variable, depending on extent of injury
IV. Hyphema—hemorrhage into the anterior chamber (see Figs. 9-12 and A-1)
  A. General
       1. Uncomplicated hemorrhage is benign.
         a) Blood is inoccuous to the structures in the anterior chamber.
         b) The blood is removed through the drainage angle.
         c) In experiments, blood placed in the anterior chamber completely clears within 48 hours.
       2. Continual bleeding results in prolonged hyphema.
         a) The blood enters and exits the chamber constantly.
         b) The color remains bright red.

      c) Under quiet rest states, cells will gravitate to the dependent part of the anterior chamber.
3. Blood changes color from bright red to dark brown or black.
      a) Indicative of clotting and degradation of RBCs
      b) Degradation products of blood may precipitate on the cornea, staining it dark (eight-ball hemorrhage).
      c) Fibrin and clot formation may result in secondary glaucoma.
4. Evidence that blood cells are not removed through the iris is substantial.
5. Fibrinolysin is released from the surface of the iris via the iridal vessels.

B. Etiologies
1. Trauma
2. Surgery
3. Spontaneous hemorrhage due to other ocular disease (i.e., collie eye anomaly)
4. Coagulopathies
      a) Spontaneous (i.e., platelet abnormalities)
      b) Toxins—overdose of anticoagulants
      c) Systemic disease—thrombocytopenia
5. Rapidly-growing neoplasms
6. Uveitis
7. Overzealous restraint
8. Vascular fragility

C. Clinical signs
1. Blood in anterior chamber—incomplete or complete
2. Acute—bright red
3. Chronic—darker, almost black
4. Obstruction to examining structures within anterior segment
5. Blood may settle to the dependent portion of the anterior chamber.
      a) Results in owner's complaint of "coming and going"
      b) When the animal is at rest, the red cells settle out.
      c) When the animal is excited and active, blood is distributed in aqueous, causing a complete red appearance.
6. Blood staining of cornea
7. Rarely, glaucoma due to angle obstruction

D. Diagnosis
1. By observation
2. History

E. Treatment—extremely controversial
1. Principles
      a) Identify the cause; this may be difficult.
      b) Prevent sequella of hyphema and rebleeding.
      c) There is little evidence that the natural course of healing of injured tissue is altered by any known therapy.

2. Corticosteroids
   a) Uncomplicated—contraindicated
   b) Presence of uveitis
      (1) Associated with chronic hyphema
      (2) Indicated topically
3. Miotics
   a) Improves facility of outflow
   b) Increases iris surface, inhibiting coagulation or clotting of cells in anterior chamber
   c) Should be used in acute hyphema
      (1) 1% pilocarpine bid or tid
      (2) For the first 48 to 72 hours
4. Mydriatics/cycloplegics
   a) May be contraindicated if the drainage angle is compromised
   b) Used in chronic hyphema with uveitis
      (1) 1% atropine SO_4 bid or tid
      (2) Check intraocular pressures
5. Cage rest
   a) Keep quiet
   b) Keep away from other animals
F. Prognosis
   1. Uncomplicated—excellent
   2. Complicated—guarded to grave
V. Iris atrophy (Fig. 1-3)
   A. Primary iris atrophy (senile iris atrophy)
      1. Observed in cats and dogs
         a) Siamese
         b) Poodles
         c) Miniature schnauzers
         d) Chihuahuas
         e) Others
      2. Etiology—unknown
      3. Clinical signs
         a) Observed in older cats and is progressive
         b) Crypts and holes become obvious
         c) Tapetal reflection may be visible through iridal defect
         d) Pupil still constricts
         e) Vision is unimpaired
      4. Diagnosis—by observation
      5. Treatment—none
      6. Prognosis—excellent
   B. Secondary iris atrophy
      1. Etiology
         a) Usually due to anterior uveitis
         b) Chronic glaucoma

         c) Trauma
    2. Clinical signs—similar to those for primary iris atrophy
    3. Diagnosis
         a) History of predisposing disease
         b) Signs of uveitis
    4. Treatment
         a) If inactive—none
         b) Treat prevailing disease
    5. Prognosis—good to grave
VI. Neoplasms of the anterior uvea
    A. Classification
        1. Primary
           a) Cell origin
              (1) Ciliary epithelium
                  i) Benign
                      (A) Adenoma
                      (B) Medulloepithelioma
                      (C) Teratoid medulloepithelioma
                  ii) Malignant
                      (A) Adenocarcinoma
                      (B) Medulloepithelioma
                      (C) Teratoid medulloepithelioma
                (2) Melanocytes
                  i) Benign
                      (A) Iris freckles—increased pigment within existing cells
                      (B) Iris nevus—increased number of pigmented cells
                  ii) Malignant melanoma
                      (A) Callenders' classification—in order of decreasing malignancy
                          (1) Epitheloid cells
                          (2) Mixed (spindle and epitheloid)
                          (3) Spindle b cells
                          (4) Spindle a cells
                      (B) The biologic activity of ocular melanomas is not as severe as in humans.
                        (1) Cats—diffuse iridal melanomas (Fig. 9-16)
                          (a) I have watched diffuse melanomas for more than 5 years in three cats without apparent metastasis
                          (b) Some authors believe these eyes should be enucleated as soon as malignant melanoma is diagnosed.
                          (c) Recent evidence in humans suggests increased metastasis following surgery.

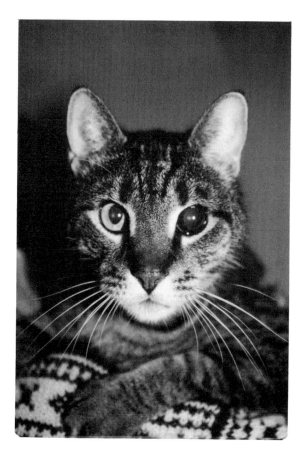

Fig. 9-16. Nine-year-old DSH male with diffuse iridal melanoma. The lesion had been present for more than 4 years with no adverse effects.

     (2) Focal epibulbar and iridal or ciliary body lesions have been excised with better than 3-year postoperative remission.

     (3) I believe metastasis is rare in dogs and cats.

  2. Secondary—except for lymphosarcoma, relatively rare but many have been reported in the anterior segment

   a) Lymphosarcoma—most common in dogs and cats

   b) Metastatic carcinomas from

    (1) Kidney

    (2) Mammary gland

    (3) Thyroid

    (4) Pancreas

    (5) Nasal cavity

    (6) Uterus

   c) Metastatic neoplasms from muscle

 B. Clinical signs

      1. Primary neoplasms
        a) Focal enlargement—distorting involved tissue
          (1) Pigmented
          (2) Nonpigmented
        b) Early lesions—noninflammatory
        c) Older, larger lesions—signs of anterior uveitis
        d) Leukocoria
        e) Secondary glaucoma—less common than reported in textbooks
      2. Secondary neoplasms—usually presented because of anterior uveitis (see Anterior uveitis)
  C. Diagnosis
      1. Clinical signs
      2. Complete physical and laboratory examination
      3. Aqueous centesis and cytology
      4. Biopsy
        a) Lymph node
        b) Ocular mass
        c) Other involved organs
  D. Treatment—depends on severity and biologic activity
      1. Primary melanoma
        a) Epibulbar melanoma—excisional biopsy early
        b) Focal lesions of iris or ciliary body—iridocyclectomy early
        c) Large masses dictate enucleation after determining possible metastasis
      2. Primary adenoma and adenocarcinoma—enucleation following survey for metastasis
      3. Metastatic neoplasms
        a) A complete oncologic workup is necessary.
        b) The extent of the primary neoplasm must be determined before ocular surgical intervention.
        c) Chemotherapy is directed to the primary neoplasm (i.e., lymphosarcoma).
        d) Symptomatic therapy is given for secondary uveitis.
  E. Prognosis
      1. Small or focal primary melanomas—good to fair
      2. Primary intraocular neoplasia with no evidence of metastasis—good to fair
      3. All others—guarded to grave

Posterior Uvea

Diseases of the choroid are discussed under Diseases of the retina.

SUGGESTED READINGS

Peiffer RL Jr (ed): Comparative Ophthalmic Pathology. Charles C. Thomas, Spring-field, IL, 1983

Slatter DH: Fundamentals of Veterinary Ophthalmology. W.B. Saunders, Phila-delphia, 1981

10

Glaucoma

ANATOMY AND PHYSIOLOGY

The general anatomy of the secretory body (Ch. 9) is important in understanding the dynamics of aqueous production and its removal, which is necessary to diagnose and treat glaucoma effectively. Aqueuous is produced both actively and passively. Passive production is by filtration, ultrafiltration, osmosis, and diffusion. Active production is by the ciliary process epithelium and its complex enzyme systems. Active secretion requires integrity of the tight junctions between the pigmented and nonpigmented epithelium. When inflammatory disease compromises these junctions, active secretions decrease and passive production increases, resulting in flare, other signs of anterior uveitis, and decreased intraocular pressure.

Increased overall production never occurs, but the outflow path may be compromised resulting in elevated intraocular pressure. This change is evidence of active secretion, because passive production is expected to decrease against a pressure gradient.

Aqueous flows from its source into the posterior chamber, through the pupil, and into the anterior chamber. It then exits the eye via the iridocorneal angle and flows between the pectinate ligaments, behind which are the trabeculae, the longitudinal muscle attachments of the ciliary body. The trabeculae form a tight, sieve-like filter that impedes flow. The resulting resistance provides turgidity to the globe, making it optically effective. Turgidity is the overall result of inhibition to flow, active and passive production. This is also evidence of active secretion. From the trabecular spaces, aqueous moves into the collecting channels, then into the intrascleral plexus and back into the general circulation.

GLAUCOMA

I. Glaucoma is characterized by elevation of intraocular pressure sufficient to cause either temporary or permanent impairment of vision (Chandler and Grant). Normal pressure is 15 to 27 mm Hg Schiotz in the dog and cat. (The mm Hg value is found by converting the scale using the chart provided with the instrument.)

II. Classification—controversial

    A. Primary (open-angle) glaucoma—an increased intraocular pressure without antecedent ocular disease

        1. The angle appears open (Fig. 10-1).

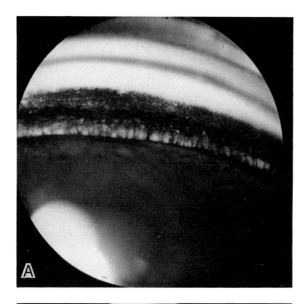

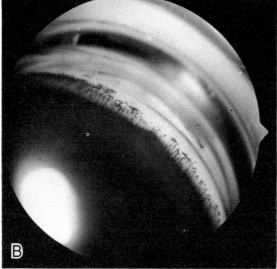

Fig. 10-1. (A) A normal angle in a normotensive dog's eye. (B) Open angle in a glaucomatous dog's eye.

2. There is no obstruction to flow through the pupil.
3. It is always bilateral.
B. Secondary glaucoma—an increased intraocular pressure with antecedent ocular disease
    1. Inflammatory debris and other sequelae to uveitis
    2. Narrow-angle—some believe this is a primary glaucoma
    3. Pupillary obstruction (see Fig. 9-14)
       a) Seclusion

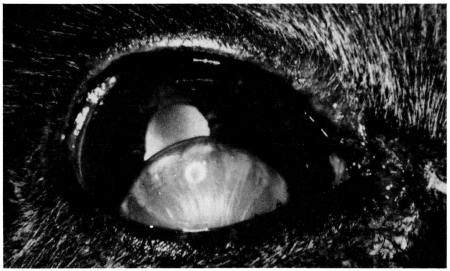

Fig. 10-2. Aged female DSH bilateral anterior lens luxation, cause unknown.

       b) Occlusion
    4. Lens-induced
       a) Anterior lens luxation (Fig. 10-2)
       b) Posterior lens luxation
         (1) Not by itself a problem
         (2) Vitreal prolapse
         (3) May be associated with other mesodermal defects
    5. Neoplastic invasion
  C. Congenital defects (Table 4-1)
    1. Animals are rarely born with glaucoma (see Fig. 9-3).
    2. Mesodermal dysgenesis (Fig. 10-3)
       a) Not clearly defined at this time
       b) Increased width of pectinate ligaments
       c) Pectinate ligament widths appears to increase as a function of aging.
       d) May predispose to glaucoma because of compromised angle
         (1) Particularly in basset hounds
         (2) Most often associated with an inflammatory component
III. Clinical signs
  A. Early—may be very subtle, but important to recognize for most effective management
    1. Increased intraocular pressure
       a) The most important diagnostic step is tonometry
       b) Cannot diagnose the disease because the eye "looks hard"

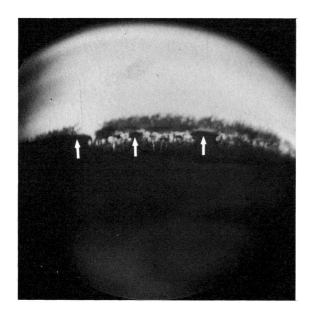

Fig. 10-3. Research bassett hound female. Goniophoto, demonstrating mesodermal dysgenesis (arrows), right eye.

      c) Schiotz tonometry is simple to perform and should be done in all practices
      d) Moderate increase—30 to 40 mm Hg
  2. Epiphora
  3. Mild blepharospasm
  4. Conjunctival hyperemia
  5. Usually no lesions demonstrable in the retina or optic nerve head
  6. Intact pupillary reflex
  7. Sight not clinically impaired
  8. Pain—subtle to absent
B. Advanced (Fig. 10-4)
  1. Markedly increased intraocular pressure (>40 mm Hg)
  2. Fixed dilated pupil
  3. Corneal opacity
      a) Striae—ruptured Descemet's membrane
      b) Edema
      c) Disruption of stromal lamellae
      d) Exposure keratopathy and associated vascularization
  4. Conjunctival and episcleral vascular congestion
  5. Buphthalmia
  6. Insensitive cornea
  7. Lens luxation or subluxation
      a) Due to stretching of the lens fibers as a result of globe enlargement
      b) Due to mesodermal dysgenesis, resulting in abnormal zonules

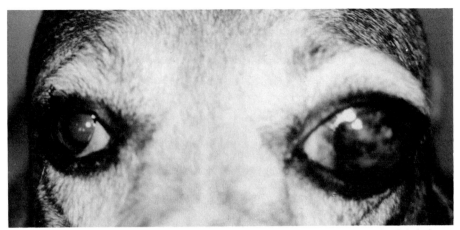

Fig. 10-4. Research bassett hound female, gross photo. Left eye demonstrates a buphthalmic eye with many of the "cardinal" signs of glaucoma. This kind of eye is not amenable to medical therapy. Goniophoto of the right eye is shown in Figure 10-5D.

      8. Blindness

      9. Gonioscopic examination (Fig. 10-5)

         a) Goniodysgenesis (see Fig. 10-5A&B)

         b) Narrow angle (see Fig. 10-5C)

         c) Cellular debris

         d) Neoplastic tissues

    10. Ophthalmoscopic examination

         a) Retinal atrophy—variable and multifocal (Fig. 10-6)

         b) Cupping of the optic nerve head

         c) Attenuation of retinal vessels

  C. Acute congestive glaucoma

      1. Most commonly observed in veterinary medicine

      2. Severe pain—often causes change in attitude

      3. All of the signs of advanced glaucoma, but accentuated

IV. Diagnosis

  A. Tonometry

      1. Digital—extremely crude; not a substitute for more effective methods (Fig. 10-7)

         a) Use proper technique—retropulsing the eye is inaccurate

         b) Place the index finger of each hand on the upper eyelid and the thumbs of each hand under the mandible (see Fig. 10-7).

         c) Apply light pressure on the globe, pressing downward and intermittently between the right and left index fingers.

         d) The pressure is determined by the ability to impress the fibrous tunic with the fingers.

      2. Indentation tonometry—Schiotz

         a) Most widely used

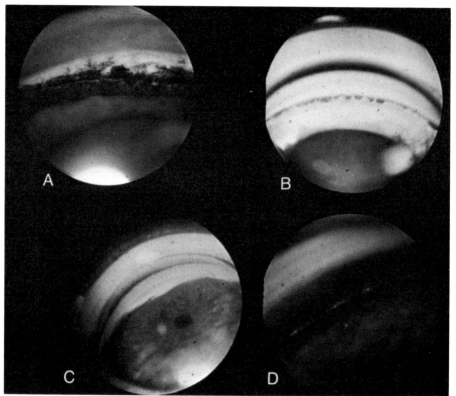

Fig. 10-5. (A) Aged Great Dane with normotensive eyes and lesions compatible with mesodermal dysgenesis. (B) Dalmation with moderately elevated (34 mm Hg, Mackay Marg) and lesions compatible with mesodermal dysgenesis. (C) Research beagle with narrow angle and elevated intraocular pressure. (D) Research bassett hound normotensive eye with mesodermal dysgenesis.

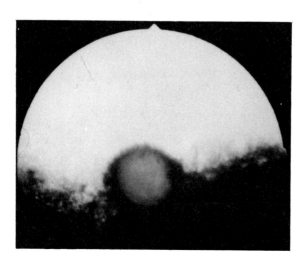

Fig. 10-6. Eight-year-old female poodle with chronic simple glaucoma and advanced retinal atrophy and optic disc "cupping."

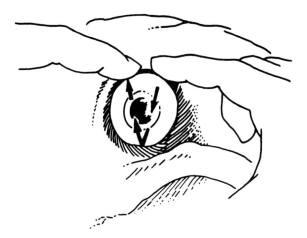

Fig. 10-7. Schematic drawing of recommended technique for digital tonometry.

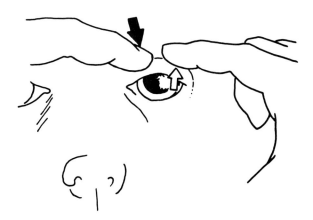

b) Convenient and relatively easy to use
c) Acceptably reliable
d) Pressure conversion charts (Friedenwald) are not designed for the dog or cat—scale readings (0 to 20) converted by the chart give results lower than the actual pressure.
e) Charts are available for the dog, but are not really necessary in my opinion. It is important to recognize that the pressure is higher than the conversion chart indicates; normal limits should be established in each practice.
f) Portable
g) Inexpensive

    h) Method—it is important to establish the technique and adhere to it
      (1) Anesthetize the cornea adequately
         i) Apply one drop of proparacaine HCl 0.5%, wait 5 minutes, then apply another drop.
        ii) The corneal reflex must be gone.
      (2) Place the animal in a dorsal recumbent position.
         i) Cradle the small animal in your arms as you would a baby.
        ii) Position the head to get the cornea of the tested eye parallel to the table.
      (3) Place the tonometer on the cornea.
         i) Keep the lids away from the footplate.
        ii) Keep the third eyelid away from the footplate.
       iii) The tonometer must be perpendicular to the corneal surface.
      (4) Three weights are commonly available—5.5 g, 7.5 g and 10 g; the weight refers to the entire weight of the instrument that rests on the cornea.
      (5) The scale on the tonometer refers to the depth of indentation.
         i) Each division on the scale is equal to 1/20 mm.
        ii) Scale readings are inversely proportional to intraocular pressure, in mm Hg.
      (6) The tonometer must be dry and clean when used; lubricants and cold sterilization solutions should not be used.
         i) After use, the instrument should be cleaned.
        ii) Use pipe cleaners to clean and dry the plunger sleeve.
       iii) Sterilization can be performed by sterilization units commercially available or gas sterilization.
      (7) Precautions
         i) Pressure should not be applied to the globe.
        ii) If the patient struggles or is restrained excessively, erroneous readings will result.
3. Applanation tonometry—electronically records (in mm Hg) the pressure necessary to flatten a 1-mm diameter of the cornea
    a) MacKay Marg (or similar type) is more accurate than Schiotz.
      (1) Electronic
      (2) Pressures are recorded on heat-sensitive paper or are digitally recorded.
      (3) Expensive
      (4) Technique must be developed
      (5) Used less often than Schiotz technique in veterinary medicine
    (b) Goldman applanation tonometry

(1) Requires a slit lamp
(2) This and modifications of it are not applicable to veterinary medicine.
B. Gonioscopy—examination of the iridocorneal angle with a contact lens placed on the anesthetized corneal surface
   1. Direct lens
      a) Examine the angle by looking directly into the angle through the lens.
      b) Use a contact solution to eliminate air bubbles between the lens and cornea.
      c) Types
         (1) Franklin—my preference (Fig. 10-8)
         (2) Cordona
         (3) Koeppe
         (4) Truncoso

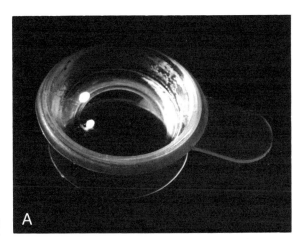

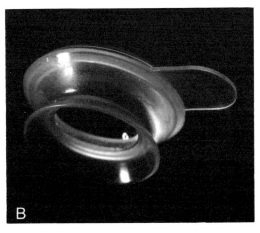

Fig. 10-8. Franklin goniolens. (A) Convex surface. (B) Concave surface, demonstrating silastic flange.

(5) Many others
2. Indirect lens
   a) Uses mirror built into the lens
   b) More difficult to develop technique and lenses are more expensive
C. Ophthalmoscopy
   1. Cupping of the optic disc (see Fig. 10-6)
   2. Retinal atrophy (see Fig. 10-6)
   3. These lesions should not be used as pathognomonic signs, but as adjunctive diagnostic criteria.
D. Tonography—determination of resistance of aqueous outflow from the anterior chamber
   1. An electronic indentation tonometry is placed on the anesthetized corneal surface for 4 minutes.
   2. Expensive
   3. Difficult to accomplish
   4. Not clinically applicable at this time
V. Treatment—depends on the type of glaucoma and recognition of the disease early in its course
A. Medical management
   1. Improve facility of outflow
      a) Sympathomimetics (adrenergic)
         (1) Epinephrine 1% to 2% sid to tid
         (2) Dipivalyl epinephrine 0.1% sid to bid—a pro drug that is a drug precursor that undergoes enzymatic reaction to the active agent within the eye
      b) Adrenergic blocking agents
         (1) Timolol maleate 0.25% to 0.50% sid to tid
         (2) Actual mechanism unknown
      c) Parasympathomimetic
         (1) Cholinergic
            i) Pilocarpine 1% to 4% sid to qid—my preference
            ii) Carbachol 0.25% to 3% sid to qid
         (2) Anticholinesterase—very toxic—must be used with extreme care
            i) Diisopropyl fluorophosphate 0.01% to 0.1% q48h to q12h
            ii) Echothiophate iodide 0.03% to 0.25% q48h to q12h
            iii) Demecarium bromide 0.125% to 0.25% q48h to q12h
   2. Decrease production
      a) Carbonic anhydrase inhibitors
         (1) Dichlorphenamide oral 5 mg/kg divided bid or tid—my preference
         (2) Acetazolamide 20 mg/kg divided bid
            i) Oral

       ii) Parenteral
      (3) Ethoxzolamide oral 4 mg/kg divided bid
      (4) Methazolamide oral 10 mg/kg divided bid
   b) Adrenergic blocking agents—timolol maleate (see above)
   c) Adrenergic agents—see above
   d) Parasympathomimetics (cholinergic)—primarily used to improve outflow, but also decrease production (see above)
  3. Reduce intraocular volume
   a) Osmotically withdraws fluid primarily from vitreous
   b) Requires an intact blood vitreous barrier
   c) Agents
      (1) Mannitol 1 to 2 g/kg IV
      (2) Glycerine 1 to 2 g/kg oral
         i) Often causes gastroenteritis
         ii) Less effective than mannitol
  4. Combinations of drugs and their effects
 B. Surgical management
  1. To preserve sight and globe (see Suggested Readings)
   a) Cyclocryosurgery—probably the best treatment available
   b) Filtering procedures—6 to 12 months is the best I have been able to obtain for control
      (1) Iridencleisis
      (2) Cyclodialysis
   c) Iridectomy
      (1) Used for secondary glaucoma due to posterior synechiae (iris bombé)
      (2) Should be a peripheral iridectomy
  2. To eliminate pain and for cosmesis
   a) Intrascleral prosthesis (see Suggested Readings)
   b) Enucleation
VI. Prognosis
 A. Depends on the stage at which the disease is presented
  1. Early—good for control
  2. Advanced—grave for control
 B. Depends on cause (i.e., primary or secondary)
  1. Primary glaucoma—not curable, can only be controlled if diagnosed early
  2. Secondary glaucoma—depends on the predisposing lesion(s)

SUGGESTED READINGS

Brightman AH, Magrane WG, Huff RW, Helper LC: Intraocular prosthesis in the dog. JAAHA 13:481, 1977

Gelatt KN (ed): Veterinary Ophthalmology. 1st Ed. Lea and Febiger, Philadelphia, 1981

Vainisi SJ: The diagnosis and therapy of glaucoma. p. 453. In Aguirre G (ed): Veterinary Clinics of North America. Vol. 3. W.B. Saunders, Philadelphia, 1973

11

The Retina and Optic Nerve

ANATOMY AND PHYSIOLOGY

The innermost of the three concentric tunics is the retina. This most complex structure is analogous to the film in a camera. The retina is derived from the forebrain and is similar to it morphologically and physiologically. It sends impulses to the visual cortex via the optic nerve, chiasm, optic tracts, and lateral geniculate body. The optic nerve, an extension of the retina, is composed of the axons of the ganglion cell layer of the retina. It is one of the first structures to appear in the developing eye, preceding even the development of the vascular and fibrous tunics.

The 10 layers of the retina, from outermost inward, are: retinal pigment epithelium (RPE); receptor layer (rods and cones); external limiting membrane; outer nuclear layer; outer plexiform layer; inner nuclear layer; inner plexiform layer; ganglion cell layer; nerve fiber layer; and internal limiting membrane. The retina is adjacent to Bruch's membrane and the choriocapillaris posteriorly and the vitreous internally. The choroid supplies nutrients to the outermost layers of the retina without retinal invasion by choroidal vessels.

The RPE in domestic animals is modified, compared with the RPE in humans. The cells overlying the tapetum are devoid of pigment, while those in the non-tapetal fundus are heavily pigmented. Clinically this is important because light is not impeded from reaching the tapetum, while that directed to the nontapetal retina is absorbed by the pigment. I believe that this provides a "macular" effect in tapetal eyes. The retina overlying the tapetum is stimulated by the most effective wavelengths in the visual spectrum, those reflected from the tapetum, giving the receptors a "double-dose" stimulation. Visual stimuli to the tapetal fundus are those originating in the ventral field, the area the animal most often uses for hunting and other visual functions. In contrast, stimuli from the dorsal field, the one that radiates sunlight, are absorbed by the heavy pigment of the RPE and underlying choroidal pigment.

An additional clinically significant characteristic is the loose attachment between the RPE and the remaining nine retinal layers. Embryologically, the invagination of the optic vescicle results in the optic cup, a two-layered neural ectodermal structure, without firm attachment between the layers. This arrangement—the tendency of the retina to separate between the RPE and the photoreceptors (retinal detachment)—persists throughout life.

The outer segments of the receptors are embedded in the RPE. The RPE phagocytize the outer rod discs as they are produced and subsequently shed. In addition, the RPE is complexly associated with the biochemical events of the photoreceptors' response to light.

The receptors are extremely complex structures. The rods have high sensitivity (sensitive to low levels of illumination) and low visual discrimination, and the cones have low sensitivity and high visual discrimination (e.g., the ability to identify print on paper). Domestic animals have rod-rich retinas, resulting in visual function different from that in primates. They function best in dim light and can interpret movement better than they can discriminate detail.

The rods are most plentiful. They have inner and outer segments. The inner segments are elongated with stacks of disc-like structures forming their outer segments, which are embedded in the RPE.

Cones are less plentiful than rods; however, an area temporal to the disc, the area centralis, has the highest cone concentration. The cones are characterized by their plump inner segments, with tapered outer segments that do not reach, but narrow toward, the RPE.

Summation, observed in all rod-rich retinas, also detracts from visual discrimination. This can be appreciated structurally in the layers of the retina. The number of receptors that converge on each ganglion cell reflects the summation phenomonen. The ratio of receptors to ganglion cells in the cat's retina is approximately 130:1.

The external limiting membrane represents the terminal bars, connecting the cell membranes of Müller cells, rods, and cones. This is a part of the "retinal scaffold" provided by Müller's cells as they extend from external to the internal limiting membranes through nine layers of the retina.

The outer nuclear layer (receptor nuclei), the thickest layer, is composed of rod and cone nuclei and connecting fibers that join them to the inner segments. The outer plexiform layer is composed of the axons of the receptor nuclei and the dendrites of the inner nuclear layer.

The inner nuclear layer (bipolar nuclei) is a composite of four types of nuclei: bipolar, amacrine, horizontal, and Müller cell. The amacrine and horizontal cells are lateral communicating cells.

The inner plexiform layer is composed of the axons of the bipolar, amacrine, and horizontal cells and the dendrites of the ganglion cells. The lateral connections in this layer provide coordination and integration of retinal function.

The ganglion cell layer in dogs and cats is relatively sparse, compared with the other nuclear layers. It is composed of cell bodies of the ganglion cell and some glial cells. Ganglion cell axons extend from the cell body to form the nerve fiber layer of the retina. The axons are nonbranching, surrounded by fibrous astrocytes and Müller cell processes. All of the fibers extend centripetally to form the optic disc. They are unmyelinated in cats until they pass through the lamina cribrosa. In dogs, they have variable degrees of myelination just anterior to and rostral to the lamina, this produces the variable configuration of the optic disc in dogs. The retinal vessels are found in this layer in dogs and cats. The retinal vascular supply in these animals has been classified as holangiotic, which implies that the whole retina is supplied by cilioretinal or central retinal arteries. Dogs and cats have cilioretinal arteries rather than a central retinal arterial supply.

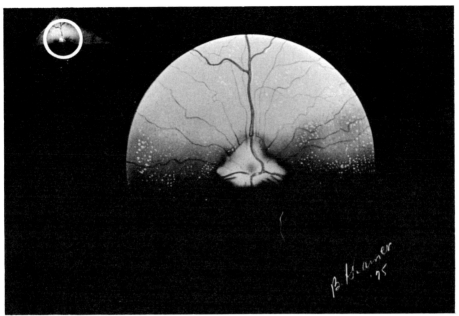

Fig. 11-1. A normal dog's fundus. Insert demonstrates approximate size of an examining field and size and primary configuration of the dog's tapetum.

The internal limiting membrane is formed by the inner termination of Müller cell processes. It covers the entire retina, except the area over the optic disc. A basement membrane secreted by the Müller and glial cells covers this structure. On ophthalmoscopic examination, this "glassy membrane" can be seen, particularly in the nontapetal retina, as a shimmering reflexion; this interesting phenomonon is useful in determining presence or absence of lesions.

The optic nerve is composed of the axons of the ganglion cells. There are two types of fibers: visual fibers, which synapse in the lateral geniculate body, and pupilomotor fibers, which synapse in the pretectal area (Fig. 1-2). The optic nerve is divided into the intraocular, orbital, and intracranial portions.

The intraocular portion basically is represented as the disc (also called papilla and nerve head). The dog has a variable configuration because of the myelination described above. The disc is elevated and usually has a prominent physiologic depression, the remnant of the hyaloid system (Fig. 11-1). The cat disc has a large physiologic depression and, unlike that of the dog, is not myelinated anterior to the lamina cribrosa. This can be observed on ophthalmoscopic examination as a deep disc with a "chicken-wire" surface. The dog has well-defined vessels on the surface of the disc; the cat does not.

The orbital portion of the optic nerve is surrounded by the meninges. The dura mater is external to the arachnoid and the pia mater the innermost. The dura provides the periorbita and orbital periosteum (Ch. 1).

The intracranial portion of the optic nerve extends from the rostral portion of the optic foramen to the optic chiasm, where the right and left nerve join and decussate variably, depending on binocularity. In dogs, 75% of the optic nerve fibers cross to the contralateral side at the chiasm; in cats, 65% to 70% of these fibers cross.

DISEASES OF THE RETINA

I. Inherited or congenital
  A. Retinal dysplasia (Fig. 11-2 and see Table 4-1)
    1. Etiologies
      a) Infection
        (1) Pregnant queen or neonate with panleukopenia virus
        (2) Experimentally in cats infected with FelV
        (3) Canine herpesvirus
        (4) Canine adenovirus
      b) Other, less important, causes
        (1) Irradiation
        (2) Nutritional deficiency (i.e., hypovitaminosis A)
        (3) Intrauterine trauma
        (4) Medication (e.g., antiviral drugs)
      c) Inherited in some dogs
        (1) Simple recessive—confirmed or presumed
          i) American cocker spaniel
          ii) Beagle
          iii) Bedlington terrier
          iv) English springer spaniel (see Fig. 11-2A&B)
          v) Labrador retriever—three forms, which may be variable expressions of the same disease
            (A) Early onset—6- to 8-week-old puppies
            (B) Associated with skeletal dysplasia
            (C) Multifocal dysplasia—first observed in 2-month- to 10-year-old dogs
          vi) Sealyham terrier
    2. Clinical signs—variable
      a) Ophthalmoscopic signs
        (1) Retinal streaks
          i) Linear hyperreflective tapetal streaks
          ii) Focal, peripapillar atapetal areas simulating postinflammatory disease (see Fig. 11-2A)
          iii) Linear gray or white streaks in the nontapetal retina
        (2) Retinal detachment—complete or partial
        (3) Intraocular hemorrhage
      b) Nystagmus

 c) Leukocoria
  (1) Retinal detachment
  (2) Cataract
 d) Blindness
3. Diagnosis

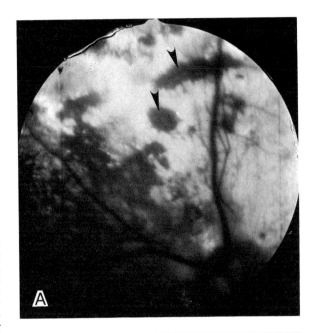

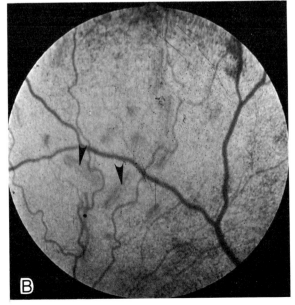

Fig. 11-2. (A) Two-year-old female English springer spaniel with bilateral retinal dysplasia. Arrows identify focal areas of dysplasia, depicted as brown atapetal zones bordered by a green band, which are surrounded by the normal yellow tapetal coloration. (B) Eight-month-old male English springer spaniel with subtle retinal dysplasia. Arrows identify linear defects, demarcated by a green color, surrounded by the normal yellow-green tapetal coloration. The center of these lesions often demonstrates hyperrelectivity.

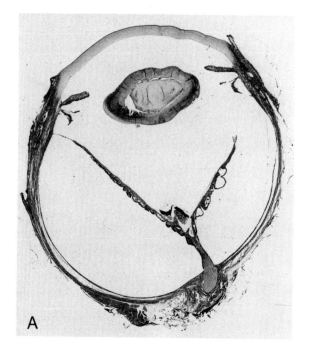

Fig. 11-3. Photomicrograph of dysplastic retina from a chocolate Labrador retriever male puppy who presented blind with bilateral retinal detachments. (A) Cross-section of globe demonstrating lesions.

      a) Clinical signs
      b) Histologic confirmation (Fig. 11-3)
         (1) Retinal folds and rossettes
         (2) Retinal detachment
    4. Treatment
      a) In general, no therapy
      b) Recommend not using animals in breeding program
    5. Prognosis
      a) Severe lesions—guarded
      b) Minor lesions—excellent for sight
B. Progressive retinal atrophy (PRA) (Fig. 11-4 and see Table 4-1)
    1. General
      a) A broad group of diseases causing similar clinical signs
      b) Differs in:
         (1) Age of onset
         (2) Rate of progression
      c) Categorized according to time of onset and rate of progression
         (1) Early onset, rapidly progressive
         (2) Early onset, slowly progressive
         (3) Late onset, slowly progressive
      d) Biochemical and morphologic defects result in lesions causing clinical signs

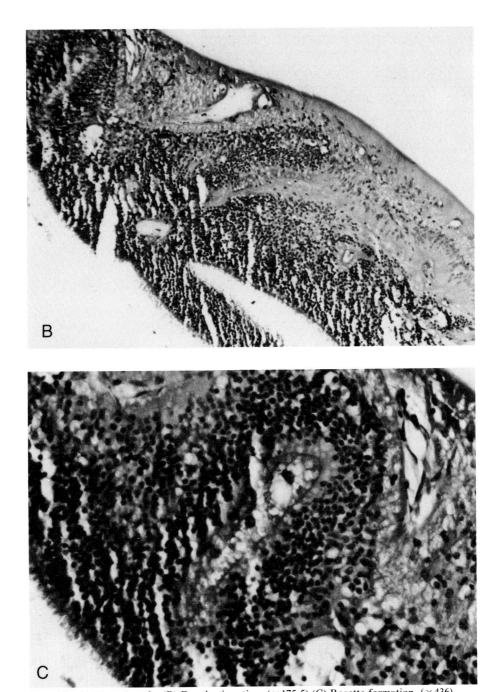

Fig. 11-3 (*continued*). (B) Dysplastic retina. ($\times 175.5$) (C) Rosette formation. ($\times 436$)

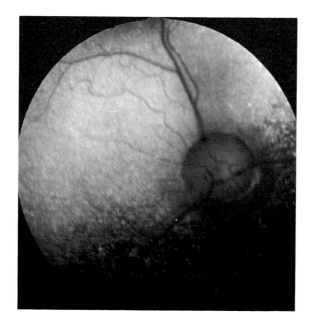

Fig. 11-4. Ten-month-old Irish setter with early progressive retinal atrophy confirmed by clinical signs, ERG, and histopathology. There was evidence of tapetal hyperreflectivity and attenuation of retinal vasculature.

       (1) Cyclic GMP increases due to lack of enzyme activator (calmodulin) and other idiopathic pathways

       (2) Microscopic and ultrastructural abnormalities of receptors

    e) Most can be identified by electrophysiologic examination (ERG)

2. Etiology

    a) Inherited by an autosomal recessive gene in all breeds studied

    b) Apparent or presumed autosomal recessive gene in all others reported

3. Predisposed breeds

    a) Early onset, rapidly progressive (onset to blind, <1 year)

       (1) Collie

       (2) Irish setter

       (3) Cardigan corgi

    b) Early onset, slowly progressive (onset <1 year of age, blind by 2 years of age)

       (1) Miniature schnauzer

       (2) Norwegian elkhound—may be two distinct diseases

    c) Late onset, slowly progressive (onset >2 years of age, blind by 4 years of age)

       (1) Afghan hound

       (2) Border collie

       (3) Cocker spaniel—English and American

       (4) Collie

       (5) Dachshund

     (6) English springer spaniel
     (7) Gordon setter
     (8) Labrador retriever
     (9) Miniature poodle
     (10) Poodle
     (11) Saluki
     (12) Samoyed
     (13) Shetland sheepdog
     (14) Cross breeds
  4. Clinical signs—always a bilateral disease
   a) Early signs
     (1) Decreased vision in dim light (nyctalopia)
     (2) Minor fundus changes
      i) Attenuation of smallest caliber vessels
      ii) Subtle changes in tapetal reflectivity
     (3) Abnormal ERG
      i) Decreased amplitude
      ii) Increased implicit times
   b) Progressive signs
     (1) Progressive nyctalopia
     (2) More attenuation of retinal vasculature
     (3) Increased tapetal reflectivity
     (4) Slightly pale optic disc
     (5) Sluggish pupillary response—poor clinical sign, but must be used as an ancillary, not pathognomonic, sign
     (6) ERG—progressive amplitude depression
   c) Advanced signs
     (1) Nyctalopia progresses to complete blindness
     (2) Complete (apparent) retinal vascular attenuation
     (3) Pallor and atrophy of the optic disc
     (4) Generalized tapetal hyperreflectivity
     (5) Animal manifests a "dumb" blind appearance
     (6) ERG—extinguished
  5. Treatment—none
  6. Prognosis
   a) Grave
     (1) Blindness is inevitable
     (2) When diagnosed in early stages, I inform the client that complete blindness will occur within 6 to 18 months
   b) Hereditary predisposition dictates exclusion of affected dogs or carriers from breeding colonies
 C. Central progressive retinal atrophy (CPRA) (Slatter's progressive retinal degeneration PRD type II—see Suggested Readings and Table 4-1)
  1. General

      a) More common in the United Kingdom than in the United States

      b) Occurs in older animals

      c) Does not usually cause complete blindness

      d) Specific retinal pigment epithelial dystrophy

         (1) Becomes hypertrophied and hyperplastic

         (2) Causes secondary cone degeneration

      e) I am not convinced that all of the reported breeds had CPRA, but rather retinal dysplasia.

  2. Breed predisposition

      a) Most common in Shetland sheepdog in my practice

      b) Reported in the following breeds:

         (1) Labrador retriever

         (2) Golden retriever

         (3) Border collie

         (4) Irish setter

         (5) English springer spaniel

         (6) Redbone coonhound

  3. Clinical signs

      a) Always bilateral

      b) Usually no signs until the animal is older than 2 years

      c) Central vision defective—the animal can't see stationary objects but can see moving objects

      d) Ophthalmoscopic examination

         (1) Distinct pigment clumping most obvious in tapetal peripapillar retinal area

         (2) Spreads centrifugally

         (3) Late in the disease

           i) Moderate attenuation of retinal vessels

           ii) Increased tapetal reflectivity

           iii) Pallor of optic disc

      e) Both day and night vision are decreased, but rarely does the animal become blind

  4. Diagnosis

      a) Clinical signs

      b) ERG—not helpful in early disease

      c) Fluorescein angiography—demonstrates defects in the RPE— client should be referred to an ophthalmologist

  5. Treatment—none

  6. Prognosis—good, but animals should not be used for breeding

D. Hereditary retinal degeneration of cats (see Table 4-1)

  1. Reported only in two litters of Persian kittens

      a) Early onset

      b) Presumed autosomal recessive

      c) I have never diagnosed the condition

  2. Clinical signs

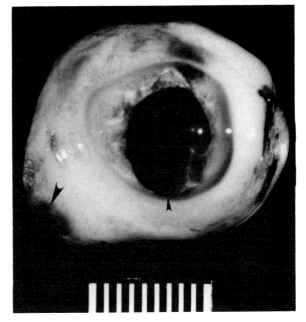

Fig. 11-5. Australian shepherd puppy's eye. Large arrow identifies equatorial staphyloma; small arrow identifies an iris coloboma. The eye was smaller than normal, and the retina was dysplastic. This is considered a multiple ocular anomaly.

       a) Nyctalopia, progressing to complete blindness
       b) Generalized tapetal hyperreflectivity
       c) Pallor of optic disc
       d) ERG
           (1) Early—depressed
           (2) Late—extinguished
       e) Pupillary areflexia
    3. Diagnosis
       a) Must be differentiated from acquired retinal atrophy
       b) Ophthalmoscopic examination
       c) ERG
    4. Treatment—none
    5. Prognosis
       a) Sight—grave
       b) These animals make good pets.
       c) These animals should not be used for breeding.
  E. Multiple ocular anomalies (Fig. 11-5 and Fig. 8-2)
    1. General
       a) Nondistinct, group resulting in controversy for categorization
       b) Usually associated with a color dilution factor (i.e., merle or white animals)
       c) Often associated with deafness
       d) Extremely variable ocular expression

e) Transmitted as an autosomal recessive gene
  (1) Confirmed in Australian shepherds
  (2) Presumed in all other breeds
2. Breed predisposition—color-dilute dogs
  a) Australian shepherd
  b) Collie—may be associated with cyclic neutropenia
  c) Dalmatian
  d) Great Dane
  e) Shetland sheepdog
3. Clinical signs—bilateral but not necessarily symmetric
  a) Gross examination
    (1) Usually a small, deformed eye
    (2) Cataracts
    (3) Heterochromia—not always pathologic
    (4) Correctopia
    (5) Iridal colobomata
    (6) Blindness or reduced vision
    (7) Deafness
  b) Ophthalmoscopic examination
    (1) Retinal detachment
    (2) Multiple colobomata and/or staphylomata
    (3) Intraocular hemorrhage
  c) Histology
    (1) Retinal dysplasia, resulting in rosette formation
    (2) Mesodermal coats are poorly developed
      i) Erratic distribution
      ii) Focal hypoplasia or aplasia of choroid, including tapetum, and sclera
    (3) Cataract
    (4) Hypoplasia of the iris and iridocorneal angle
4. Diagnosis
  a) By observation and anamnesis
  b) Ophthalmoscopic examination
  c) Histologic confirmation
5. Treatment—none
6. Prognosis
  a) Animals with this condition frequently have concomitant problems and make poor pets.
  b) When the disease has minimal expressitivity, the animals make acceptable pets.
  c) The animal should not be used for breeding.
F. Stationary night blindness (congenital nighblindness) (see Table 4-1)
  1. General
    a) Not confirmed in small animals (see Suggested Readings)
    b) Possible category for further investigation

      c) Three breeds that do not completely fall into the typical progressive retinal atrophy (PRA) pattern suggest this possibility.

      d) Definitive inheritability is unknown, but it appears as an autosomal recessive gene.

  2. Breed predisposition

      a) Briard

      b) Tibetan terrier

      c) Miniature schnauzer—may be early onset, slowly progressive

  3. Clinical signs

      a) Normal day vision

          (1) Stationary nyctalopia has not been established

          (2) May develop hemeralopia later on

      b) Early-onset nightblindness (younger than 6 months)

      c) No well-defined retinal lesions

          (1) Hazy gray tapetal reflex in very young puppies (?)

          (2) Tapetal granularity (?)

      d) ERG

          (1) Loss or decreased amplitude of b wave

          (2) Increased implicit time in light-adapted eyes

      e) Histology

          (1) No demonstrable abnormalities

          (2) No information available for older dogs

  4. Diagnosis

      a) Clinical signs

      b) ERG

  5. Treatment—none

  6. Prognosis

      a) These animals make acceptable pets.

      b) The animals shoud not be used for breeding stock.

G. Hemeralopia (see Table 4-1)

  1. General

      a) Relatively rare

      b) Early onset

      c) Transmitted by an autosomal recessive gene

  2. Breed predisposition

      a) Alaskan malamute—only confirmed breed

      b) Miniature poodle—presumed

  3. Clinical signs

      a) Day vision absent—demonstrable at 2 months of age

      b) No gross ophthalmoscopic lesions

      c) Dogs dark-adapt and are sighted in dim illumination

      d) ERG

          (1) Absent photopic response

          (2) Normal scotopic response

      e) Histology

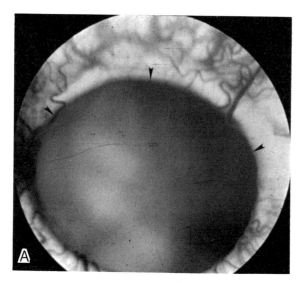

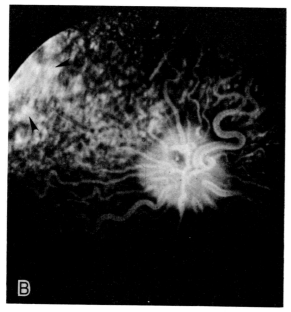

Fig. 11-6. (A) Collie stud used in our research colony (gross lesions. Fig. 11-7). Arrows identify the large scleral defect lined with choroid, which is by definition a staphyloma rather than ectasia. The "white" margin indicates an absence or diminuition of choroidal vessels, hence choroidal hypoplasia. (B) Fluorescein angiograph of a research collie female with increased tortuosity of retinal vessels. Arrows identify a choroidal hypoplastic zone.

    (1) Light-microscopic examination—normal, particularly early on
    (2) Electron-microscopic examination
        i) Early—normal
        ii) Late—degeneration of cone outer segments
4. Diagnosis

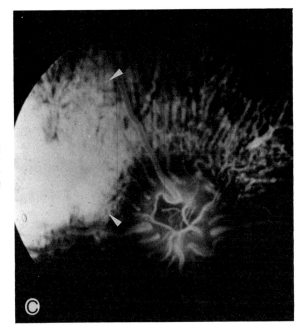

Fig. 11-6 (*continued*). (C) Fluorescein angiograph of a research collie female with choroidal hypoplasia. Arrows identify the choroidal hypoplastic region. Notice the absence of vessels.

        a) Clinical signs
        b) ERG
    5. Treatment—none
    6. Prognosis
        a) These animals make acceptable pets.
        b) The animals should not be used for breeding.
  H. Collie eye anomaly (collie ectasia syndrome) (Fig. 11-6)
    1. General
        a) One of the best-characterized inherited lesions
        b) Very widespread, but rarely causes blindness
        c) Breeders grades these lesions, but the system does not correlate
           phenotype with genotype
            (1) Grade 1—tortuous vessels (Fig. 11-6B)
            (2) Grade 2—choroidal hypoplasia (Fig. 11-6A&C)
            (3) Grade 3—peripapillar colobomata, posterior staphylomata
                (see Fig. 11-6A and Fig. 11-7)
            (5) Grade 5—intraocular hemorrhage
        d) This is a lesion of the outer layer of the developing optic cup
           resulting in abnormal mesodermal maturation.
        e) Transmitted by an autosomal recessive gene in collies and Shet-
           land sheepdogs and, presumably, in other breeds
    2. Breed predisposition
        a) Collie—rough and smooth

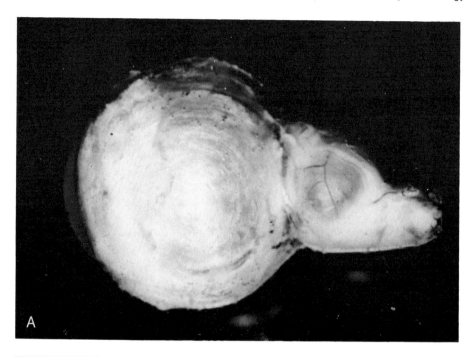

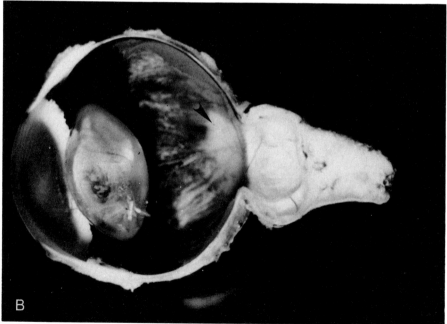

Fig. 11-7. External view gross photograph of enucleated affected eye from a research collie that was clinically sighted (Fig. 11-6A). (B) Internal view of the same eye. Arrow identifies choroidal hypoplasia seen in Figure 11-6. Compare fundus photograph with this gross photograph for orientation.

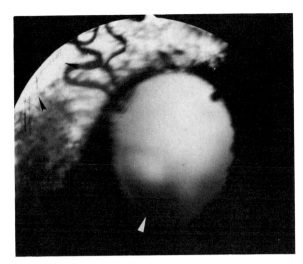

Fig. 11-8. White German shepherd male puppy, demonstrating lesions similar to the collie eye anomaly. Large arrow identifies coloboma of the optic disc area; small arrows identify choroidal hypoplasia. Vessels are tortuous. The puppy was not blind.

    b) Shetland sheepdog
    c) German shepherd (my data) (Fig. 11-8)
    d) Basenji (?)
    e) Rarely occurs in cats (Fig. 11-9)
  3. Clinical signs
    a) Vision
      (1) Blindness occurs in less than 1% of animals, according to my records.
      (2) Blindness may be unilateral or bilateral.
    b) Ophthalmoscopic appearance

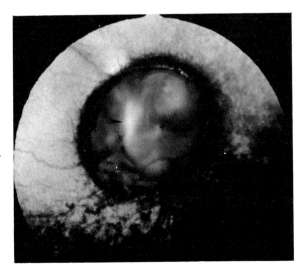

Fig. 11-9. DSH 18-month-old male demonstrating a peripapillar coloboma. Small arrow identifies to the deepest defect; large arrow identifies the next "shelf." See Figure 11-7B for a comparison of the margin of the defect. It is pigmented in this cat.

    (1) Increased retinal vascular tortuosity—not very important
    (2) Choroidal hypoplasia
        i) Most common lesion
        ii) Temporal slightly dorsal to optic disc
        iii) Variable size
        iv) Neonates (younger than 3 months) may manifest lesions that become normal in appearance as the animal matures ("go normals")
    (3) Colobomata
        i) More severe lesions but similar to choroidal hypoplasia—the absence of mesodermal development involves sclera as well as choroid
        ii) Not a lesion of the optic nerve
            (A) Peripapillar mesodermal defect
            (B) May not be immediately adjacent to disc
    (4) Retinal detachment
        i) Secondary lesion
        ii) Bullous detachment
        iii) Complete conus detachment with or without disinsertion
    (5) Intraocular hemorrhage—secondary lesion
    (6) Other lesions
        i) Vermiform streaks
            (A) Retinal folds
            (B) Usually disappear with maturation
            (C) I have not demonstrated rosettes on histologic examination.
        ii) Cataracts—I could not establish any correlation with CEA and cataracts in my colony of experimental dogs
        iii) Microphthalmia
            (A) There were no small globes by measurement in our research animals.
            (B) I believe this was incorrectly included early on in CEA research as a part of the color-dilute disease lesion (see Microphthalmia).
        iv) Corneal dystrophy—concommitant but not genetically associated
  4. Diagnosis—ophthalmoscopic examination
  5. Treatment—none
  6. Prognosis
    a) Detachments and intraocular hemorrhage—animals make poor pets
    b) Other lesions—animals make excellent pets
    c) The animal should not be used for breeding.
I. Hypoplasia/aplasia optic nerve (Fig. 11-10 and see Table 4-1)

   1. General
     a) Previously reported as a congenital, not inherited, defect
     b) Breeding trials demonstrate a definite inherited predisposition in miniature poodles—mode of inheritance unknown
     c) Clinically, may be unilateral or bilateral
     d) May be complete or partial
     e) Probably hypoplasia or aplasia of the ganglion cells
   2. Breed predisposition
     a) Beagle
     b) Miniature poodle (see Fig. 11-10B and 11-10C)
     c) Collie (?)
     d) Miniature dachshund
     e) Saint Bernard (?) (see Fig. 11-10A)
     f) Cocker spaniel (?)
   3. Clinical signs
     a) Vision
       (1) Blind
       (2) Sighted
     b) Optic nerve
       (1) Small—retinal vessels and fundus appear normal
       (2) Absent
         i) Retinal vessels absent
         ii) Retina appears dull
     c) ERG
       (1) Normal if vessels are present
       (2) Extinguished if retinal vessels are absent
     d) Pupillary reflexia—variable
   4. Diagnosis
     a) Ophthalmoscopic examination
     b) Clinical signs
   5. Treatment—none
   6. Prognosis
     a) These animals make excellent pets.
     b) These animals should not be used for breeding.
J. Miscellaneous inherited diseases
   1. Gyrate atrophy of choroid and retina (see Table 4-1)
     a) Etiology—presumed autosomal recessive in mixed breeds of cats
     b) Clinical signs
       (1) Generalized retinal atrophy
       (2) Pupillary areflexia
       (3) Extinguished ERG
     c) Diagnosis
       (1) Clinical signs
       (2) Hyperornithenemia
       (3) Ornithenuria

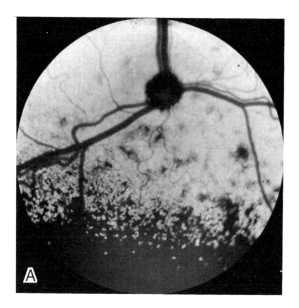

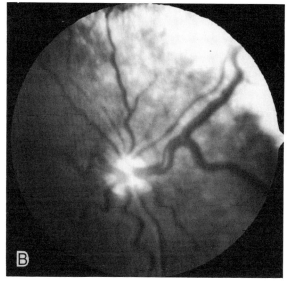

Fig. 11-10. (A) Saint Bernard male puppy with bilateral optic nerve hypoplasia. Compare disc size with that in Figure 11-1. (B) Research miniature poodle female, 10 weeks old, left eye. Puppy was not blind in either eye.

    d) Treatment—none
    e) Prognosis—grave
  2. GM gangliosidosis and other storage diseases—not primary retinal diseases (see Suggested Readings)
    a) Autosomal recessive transmission in Siamese cats
    b) Intraretinal punctate gray foci
    c) May cause blindness in advanced disease

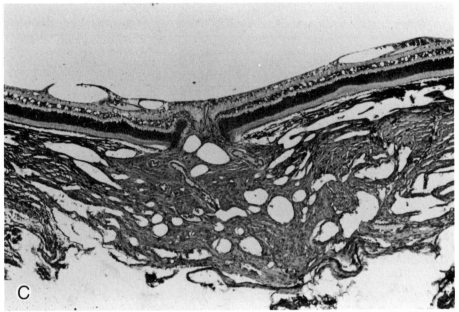

Fig. 11-10 (*continued*). (C) Histopathology of an eye from an affected research poodle. Notice the paucity of nerve fiber layer. (H & E, × 16)

II. Acquired retinal disease
  A. Nutritional or toxic retinal degeneration
    1. Taurine deficiency in cats (Fig. 11-11)
      a) Etiology—taurine-deficient diet (i.e., dog food)
      b) Clinical signs
        (1) Simulates PRA and gyrate atrophy of choroid and retina
        (2) Nyctalopia, progressing to complete blindness
        (3) Tapetal hyperreflectivity
        (4) Retinal vascular attenuation
        (5) Diminished pupillary reflexia to areflexia
        (6) Extinguished ERG
      c) Diagnosis
        (1) Clinical signs
        (2) ERG
        (3) History of diet
      d) Treatment
        (1) Late in the disease—none
        (2) Early—supplement with 1 teaspoon taurine per week divided in daily amounts or feed commercial cat food
      e) Prognosis

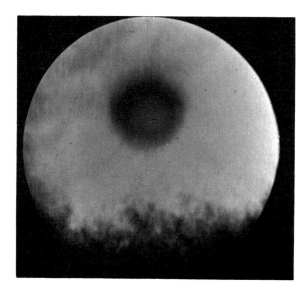

Fig. 11-11. DSH female, 2 years old, research cat on a taurine-deficient diet. Notice absence of vessels and dull appearance of optic disc. Hyperreflectivity is not well demonstrated in black and white. Cat was blind.

          (1) Advanced—grave
          (2) Early—fair to good
  2. Thyamine deficiency in cats—rare
     a) Etiology—diet of overprocessed commercial food or all-fish diet
     b) Clinical signs
          (1) Peripapillar edema
          (2) Mydriasis
          (3) Cats are not blind
          (4) Ataxic with other neurologic disorders
     c) Diagnosis
          (1) History
          (2) Clinical signs
          (3) Ophthalmoscopic examination
     d) Treatment—dietary supplementation
     e) Prognosis—excellent
  3. Other dietary deficiencies—rare
     a) Vitamin A—nyctalopia
     b) Vitamin E—degeneration of the rod and cone outer segments
  4. Retinal intoxicants
     a) General
          (1) Many agents can cause retinal degeneration.
          (2) Often tapetal-dependent
          (3) Usually a history of intoxication
     b) Agents
          (1) Zinc-chelating agents

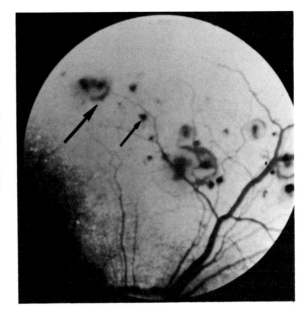

Fig. 11-12. Tapetal retina of a zinc pyridinethione-treated dog. Punctate pigmented lesions (small arrow) and bullseye lesion (large arrow) due to peripheral hemorrhage are demonstrated. Seventh day after dosing. From Cloyd, et al.

       i) Affect the tapetal cells, resulting in ischemia, retinal hemorrhage detachment, and blindness (Fig. 11-12)

       ii) Found in some human shampoos

    (2) Ketamine/methyl nitrosourea

       i) Causes blindness within 1 week after administration in experiments (Fig. 11-13)

       ii) May be important clinically if alkylating agents are present when ketamine is administered

       iii) 15 of 18 cats that received multiple injections of ketamine had signs of retinal atrophy indistinguishable from taurine-deficient retinal lesions

    (3) Others of less significance

       i) Chloraquine

       ii) Diaminodiphenozyalkanes

       iii) Ethambutol

B. Inflammatory retinal diseases

    1. General

       a) Retinal inflammation alone is rare if present at all—usually involves the choroid and sometimes involves the vitreous

        (1) Retinochoroiditis = primary retinal lesion

        (2) Chorioretinitis = primary choroidal lesion

       b) Local reactions taking place at the site of injury

       c) Ophthalmoscopic appearance is nonspecific, depending on the severity and extent of the exciting etiology

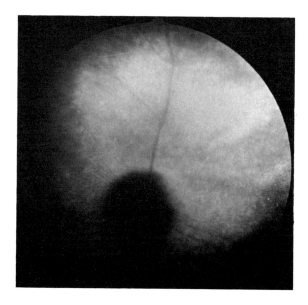

Fig. 11-13. Research DSH injected with methyl nitrosaurea and ketamine HCl. Both eyes were similarly involved. Cat was blind and ERG was flat. Ophthalmoscopically, the retinas would be affected as early as 72 hours after injection of the agents.

    d) Early inflammation—usually nonsuppurative
    e) Chronic inflammation—suppurative and, histologically, often granulomatous
    f) Many stimuli can result in an inflammatory reaction.
    g) Active (itis) and sequela (opathy) may be present.
  2. Etiologies
    a) Infectious
      (1) Bacteria
        i) Septicemia—many organisms
        ii) Brucellosis—dog (see Fig. 9-6)
        iii) Tuberculosis—cat
      (2) Virus—significant class
        i) Dogs
          (A) Canine distemper
          (B) Infectious rhinotonsillitis (?)
        ii) Cats
          (A) FelV (Fig. 11-14)
          (B) FIP (Fig. 11-15)
      (3) Fungus—dogs and cats
        i) Blastomycosis—most common in dogs (Fig. 11-16)
        ii) Cryptomycoccosis—most common in cats (Fig. 11-17)
        iii) Coccidioidomycosis—endemic in the far southwest
        iv) Histoplasmosis—endemic in the Ohio river valley (Fig. 11-18)
      (4) Protozoa
        i) Toxoplasmosis—most common in cats (see Fig. 11-17B)

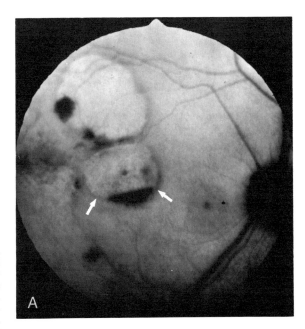

Fig. 11-14. (A) Two-year-old DSH female. FelV-related red cell aplasia, right eye. Arrows identify boat or keel hemorrhage. Notice the PCV within a vesicle-like circle. This occurs between the retina and the vitreous. (B) Three-year-old DSH male. FelV-related anemia (PCV 6.3), left eye. Arrows identify flame-shaped hemorrhage, which locates it in the nerve fiber layer of the retina.

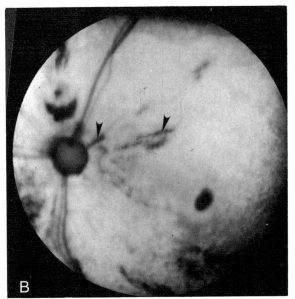

       ii) Leishmaniasis—not important in the United States
  (5) Rickettsia—ehrlichiosis in dogs
  (6) Algae—protothecosis
  (7) Parasites
       i) *Toxocara canis*—dogs

ii) Cats—see Suggested Readings
b) Trauma
(1) Proptosis
(2) Penetrating injury
(3) Surgery

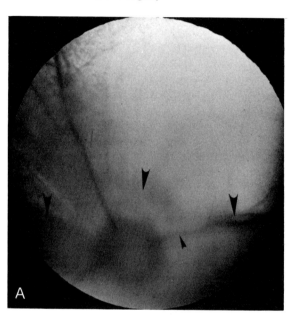

Fig. 11-15. (A) Siamese male cat, 9 years old. Feline infectious peritonitis with a proliferative detachment inferior to the optic disc. Large arrows outline detachment; small arrow identifies inflammatory reaction obliterating underlying structures. (B) Histology of the left eye of the cat in Figure 11-15A. Arrows identify protein exudate beneath the receptors, elevating the retina. (H & E, ×100)

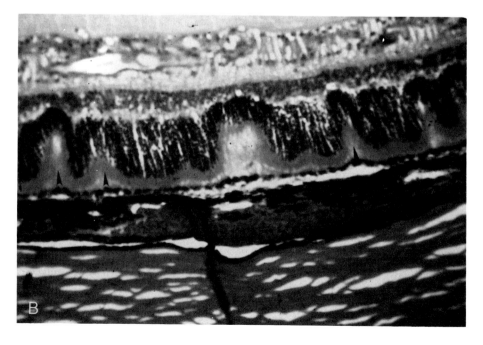

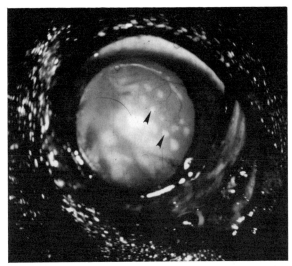

Fig. 11-16. Three-year-old Doberman pinscher male with disseminated blastomycosis, right eye. Organisms were identified intraocularly. Arrows identify inflammatory foci observed on gross examination within a detached retina.

    c) Toxins—see page 248
    d) Immune-mediated diseases
       (1) Autoimmune hemolytic anemia
       (2) SLE—see page 90
       (3) Hyperviscosity syndrome, gammopathies
       (4) Immune-mediated thrombocytopenia
       (5) Idiopathic exudative retinal detachment
       (6) VKH—see page 200
    e) Primary vascular disease
       (1) Hypertension
         i) Renal disease
         ii) Hypothyroidism
         iii) Arteriosclerosis
         iv) Adrenal neoplasia
       (2) Preretinal vascularity or arteriolar loops
    f) Nutritional—see page 247
    g) Neoplastic disease
       (1) FelV—very common
       (2) Reticulosis—pseudotumor in dogs
       (3) Lymphosarcoma—dogs
       (4) Choroidal melanoma—rare (Fig. 1-10)
       (5) Metastatic neoplasms—any neoplasm may metastasize to the eye
  3. Clinical signs
    a) Nonspecific
    b) May accompany any of the predisposing causes:
       (1) Retinitis

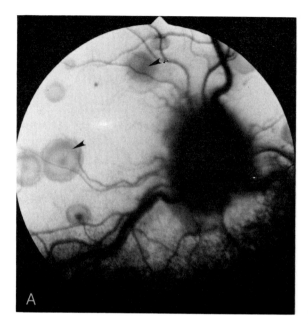

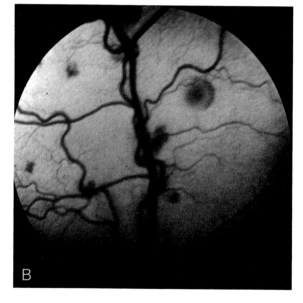

Fig. 11-17. (A) Four-year-old Siamese male cat, right eye. The cat presented with a rhinitis and pneumonia. Cytologic study confirmed the diagnosis of cryptococcosis. The cat was killed and *Cryptococcus* organisms identified histologically. Arrows identify well-circumscribed inflammatory lesions elevating the retina. Notice the apparent optic neuritis. (B) Eighteen-month-old DSH female research cat, experimentally infected with *Toxoplasma gondii*. This animal did not display any clinical signs compatible with the disease. The organisms were demonstrated in the histologic sections of the eye. Notice the similarity to Figure 11-17A.

    i) Retinal edema (thickened retina)
      (A) Decreased tapetal reflectivity
      (B) Dull nontapetal reflection
      (C) Accompanies any retinitis
      (D) Anterior retinal surface more glistening—must be

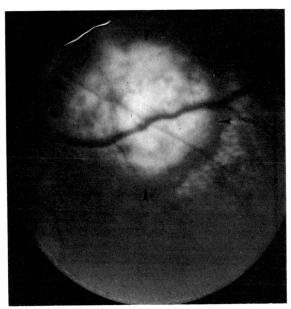

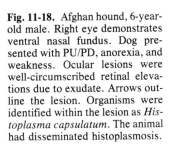

Fig. 11-18. Afghan hound, 6-year-old male. Right eye demonstrates ventral nasal fundus. Dog presented with PU/PD, anorexia, and weakness. Ocular lesions were well-circumscribed retinal elevations due to exudate. Arrows outline the lesion. Organisms were identified within the lesion as *Histoplasma capsulatum*. The animal had disseminated histoplasmosis.

differentiated from physiologic "shimmer" of young animals

ii) Exudates
   (A) Hard—solid appearance
      (1) Discrete
      (2) Smooth, distinct edges
      (3) Represent intraretinal lipoid deposits
      (4) Usually takes longer to develop than soft exudate
   (B) Soft—fuzzy appearance (cotton wool spots)
      (1) Indistinct gray patches
      (2) Larger than hard exudates
      (3) Usually develop rapidly
      (4) None are pathognomonic

iii) Hemorrhage (Fig. 11-19)
   (A) Any red patch is probably a hemorrhage
      (1) Eliminate:
         (a) Neovascularization
         (b) Choroidal vessels (i.e., atapetal retina)
      (2) Deep choroidal hemorrhage may appear black
   (B) Appearance determined by retinal structure
      (1) Flame (linear) shape—nerve fiber layer—found between parallel nerve fibers (see Fig. 11-14B)

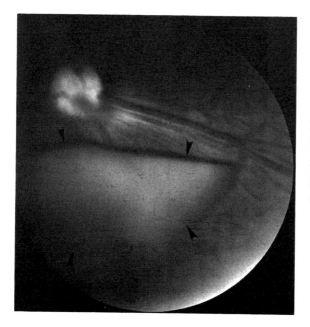

Fig. 11-19. Basenji puppy in research colony, approximately 3 weeks old, with spontaneous preretinal hemorrhage. Arrows outline the fresh hemorrhage. It was bright red and resorbed within 15 days without adverse sequelae.

(2) Müller's fibers produce "round" columns in the outer portions, resulting in small, round hemorrhages (see Fig. 11-12)

(3) Preretinal hemorrhage (see Fig. 11-19)

    (a) Blood pools between retina and vitreous face

    (b) Results in pool of blood in a round pocket

    (c) Cells gravitate to the dependent portion, which resembles the hull of a boat—called a boat hemorrhage (see Fig. 11-14A)

(C) All are nonspecific signs, but blood dyscrasias should be investigated when predominant lesion is hemorrhage

iv) Retinal vessels

(A) Elevations of vessels

    (1) Blurred appearance—direct ophthalmoscopy

        (a) More positive diopters to focus clearly

        (b) Eliminate blurring from other causes

    (2) Etiologies

        (a) Retinal detachment—gray "floating curtain"

            (i) Spontaneous retinal detachments (Fig. 11-20)

        (b) Subretinal edema

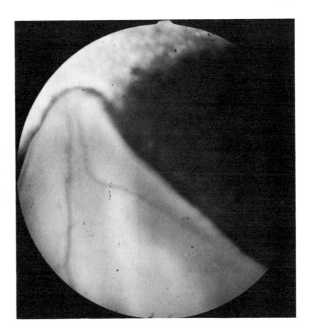

Fig. 11-20. Two-year-old dachshund male, right eye with spontaneous retinal detachment. There was no evidence of inflammatory disease. The prevalence in miniature dachshunds, dachshunds, and miniature poodles is greater than at-risk dogs, in my experience.

    (*c*) Subretinal mass—solid, fleshy appearance
        (*i*) Primary neoplasm
        (*ii*) Secondary neoplasm
    (*d*) Focal orbital mass—pushes on fibrous tunic
        (*i*) When eye moves, lesion "moves" ophthalmoscopically (see Fig. 3-13)
        (*ii*) Used to differentiate from intraocular mass and extraocular mass
(*B*) Caliber—normally in dogs and cats, vascular caliber is variable, but the arteries are approximately one-fourth the caliber of the vein
    (*1*) Enlarged
        (*a*) Impeded venous flow (i.e., papilledema)
        (*b*) Increased circulation (i.e., hypertension)
    (*2*) Decreased
        (*a*) Anemia
        (*b*) Retinal atrophy
(*C*) Color
    (*1*) Must develop skill by practice
    (*2*) Light reflex—property of the transparency and reflectiveness of vessel wall
    (*3*) Changes in vessel wall changes light reflex (i.e., copper wire effect of atrophy)

           (*4*) Increased color
              (*a*) Polycythemia
              (*b*) Hypertension
           (*5*) Decreased color
              (*a*) Anemia
              (*b*) Atrophy
           (*6*) Pink—lipemia retinalis—associated with abnormal lipid metabolism
              (*a*) Acute pancreatitis
              (*b*) Diabetes mellitus
              (*c*) Steroid therapy, especially in cats
        (*D*) Sheating of vessels—perivascular cuffing
           (*1*) Accompanies any inflammatory disease
           (*2*) Margins of the vessels are indistinct
           (*3*) Light reflex absent
    (2) Retinopathy—sequelae to retinitis. These lesions can best be understood by studying the anatomic relationship of the three concentric tunics and the 10 layers of the retina. When inflammation or degeneration results in destruction, migration, or proliferation of tissues, the ophthalmoscopic appearance changes
      i) Loss of retina, including RPE
        (*A*) Tapetal hyperreflectivity
           (*1*) Focal
           (*2*) Generalized
        (*B*) When tapetal cells are lost, a bullseye lesion results.
           (*1*) Perilesional hyperreflectivity
           (*2*) Dark (choroidal) pigment central
           (*3*) Must be differentiated from pigmented epithelial proliferation
        (*C*) Nontapetal fundus
           (*1*) Pale
           (*2*) Light brown
      ii) Pigment epithelial migration, hyperplasia, or hypertrophy
        (*A*) Pigment "clumping" overlying tapetum
        (*B*) Cobblestone effect in nontapetal retina
        (*C*) Best example is progressive central retinal atrophy
  4. Diagnosis
    a) Owner's complaint of systemic illness and/or blindness
    b) Ophthalmoscopic examination may be contributory to diagnosing systemic disease
    c) Vitreous centesis
      (1) Reserved for severe lesions; particularly useful in mycosis

        (2) Culture
        (3) Cytology
    d) Serologic examination (i.e., toxoplasmosis, blastomycosis, and
       histoplasmosis)
    e) Radiographs—chest—useful in neoplasms and mycosis
    f) Cardiovascular evaluation
    g) Immune screen
  5. Treatment
    a) Must be directed toward exciting etiology
        (1) Specific or broad-spectrum antibiotic(s)
        (2) Antifungal agents (see p. 19—Pharmacology)
        (3) Immunosuppressive agents
        (4) Antiinflammatory agents
        (5) Enucleation or exenteration if neoplastic
    b) The position (posterior uvea and retina) makes it necessary to
       medicate systemically.
  6. Prognosis—good to grave, depending on the extent of the lesion(s)

DISEASES OF THE OPTIC NERVE

  I. Colobomata of the optic nerve, as described in collies, etc., is not a lesion
     of the optic nerve as reported, but rather a lesion of the peripapillar
     mesoderm.
 II. There are few true congenital lesions of the optic nerve per se. Usually
     they are secondary to other disease (i.e., ganglion cell hypoplasia/aplasia;
     see p. 244).
III. Atrophy—sequella to retinal degenerations of many kinds
 IV. Inflammation of the optic nerve—unilateral or bilateral (Fig. 11-21)
    A. Etiologies—same as for retinitis
    B. Clinical signs
        1. Swollen optic nerve, extending vitread
        2. Dilated vessels, resulting in hyperemia
        3. Focal hemorrhage
        4. Exudates observed on and around disc
        5. Peripapillar retinal elevation
        6. Blindness
        7. Papilledema is less common and has no inflammatory component.
    C. Diagnosis
        1. History
        2. Ophthalmoscopic examination
        3. Similar diagnostic evaluation as for retinal diseases
    D. Treatment—same as for retinitis
    E. Prognosis—same as for retinitis

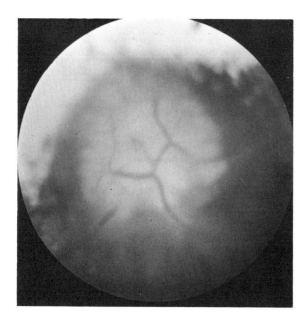

Fig. 11-21. Mixed 5-year-old male presented with an owner's complaint of blindness. The margins of the disc were indistinct due to peripapillar exudate. The disc protruded vitread. The cause was never identified.

SUGGESTED READINGS

Loew ER, Riis RC: Congenital nyctalopia in the tibetan terrier. Proc Am Coll Vet Ophthalmol 14:82, 1983

Murray JA, Blakemore WF, Barnett KC: Ocular lesions in cats with GM—gangliosidosis with visceral involvement. J Small Anim Pract 18:1, 1977

Rubin LF: Atlas of Veterinary Ophthalmoscopy. Lea & Febiger, Philadelphia, 1974

Slatter DH: Fundamentals of Veterinary Ophthalmology 1st. Ed. WB Saunders, Philadelphia, 1981

12

The Lens and Vitreous

THE LENS

Anatomy and Physiology

The lens is an asymmetric biconvex sphere with the anterior flatter than the posterior surface. The apical positions of the lens are called the anterior and posterior poles. The circumference, called the equator, is the predominant zone of attachments for the lenticular zonules. The lens capsule is weakest at the equator. The zonules attach anterior and posterior to the equator in a crossing fashion. These zonules extend to the ciliary body, and ciliary muscle contraction results in a release of tension on the zonules, permitting the lens to become more biconvex for near vision. In contrast, relaxation of the ciliary muscles increases zonular tension, resulting in flattening of the lens for distant vision. This process of "accommodation" is poorly developed in domestic animals, compared with primates.

The lens is one of the oldest structures in the eye-containing portions that were present in the embryo and fetus. The capsule stems from the basement membrane of the cuboidal cells of the embryonic lens vesicle. The anterior capsule is thicker than the posterior. Immediately under the anterior capsule is the germinal cell layer (anterior epithelium), the origin for the new fibers formed throughout the animal's life. The germinal epithelial cells migrate peripherally and elongate at the equator, with each cell extending anteriorly under the epithelium and posteriorly beneath the capsule. They meet fellow fibers in front and back in a "Y" suture pattern, which is usually right side up anteriorly and upside down posteriorly. The newer lens cells contain nuclei; as they are compressed centrally by new fibers covering them, they loose their nuclei.

The next zone is the cortex, which can be identified on histologic examination by its young lens fibers that contain nuclei. The cortex is widest at the equator and thinnest axially. The cortical lens fibers are incorporated into the adult nucleus when they loose their nuclei. The adult nucleus is the largest growth area of the lens. Immediately inside the adult nucleus is the fetal nucleus. The most inner and central zone, the embryonal nucleus, is the only nucleus that does not have a suture line. During embryonal development, elongation of the posterior cuboidal cells results in obliteration of the lumen of the optical vesicle to form the embryonal nucleus.

Continual lens growth results in a denser, less elastic lens with increasing age. The lens begins absorbing certain wavelengths, resulting in a "blue" appearance to the older animal's lens, often misdiagnosed as a cataract. This is a normal aging process.

Although the lens continues to grow and metabolize throughout life, there is no direct blood supply. Oxygen and metabolites are provided by the aqueous. Glucose is the primary source of energy. The lens capsule is not insulin-dependent, and glucose diffuses through the capsule and by assisted transport. The Embden–Myerhof pathway is the principle means of anaerobic glucose metabolism, and Krebs' cycle provides a small amount of aerobic glycolysis. Elevated glucose levels cause additional glycolysis via the sorbital shunt. This mechanism causes an alteration in osmotic tensions, resulting in imbitition of fluid by the lens.

The lens is predominantly (87%) soluble proteins (i.e., alpha-crystallin, beta-crystallin, and gamma-crystallin) and is about 12% insoluble albuminoid and has trace amounts of muco and nucleo proteins. These proteins comprise about 35% of the lens, and water contributes about 65%. Aging results in an increase concentration of insoluble albuminoid and decreased water and soluble proteins.

Diseases

  I. Congenital anomalies—extremely rare and usually associated with other
     anomalous conditions
     A. Aphakia
     B. Coloboma—probably due to a defect or lack of development of the
        zonules

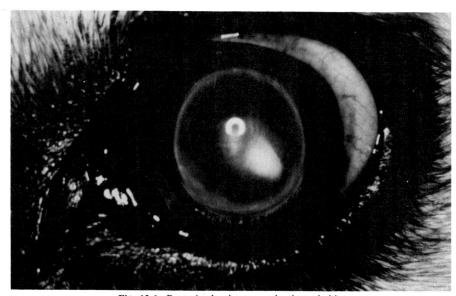

Fig. 12-1. Posterior lenticonus and spherophakia.

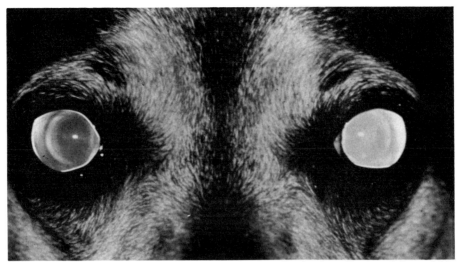

Fig. 12-2. Aged hound dog with lenticular sclerosis. Note the circular reflection of the nuclei in both eyes.

    C. Ectopia lentis—due to abnormal development or attachment of the zonules

    D. Lenticonus—cause unknown (Fig. 12-1)

        1. Posterior or anterior—posterior more common than anterior lenticonus

        2. A spherical posterior protrusion of the axial surface

        3. Histologically

            a) Posterior capsule thinned

            b) Lens cortex bulges posteriorly

            c) Cortical fibers have abnormal nuclei

 II. Lenticular sclerosis—not considered a cataract in veterinary medicine (Fig. 12-2)

    A. Normal aging process and does not require surgery or treatment

        1. Nuclear fibers become compressed, and the centermost nuclei become more dense than fibers closer to the cortex

        2. Contains less water and soluble protein—insoluble albuminoid increases

        3. Alters refractive index

    B. Lenticular sclerosis is demonstrable in dogs and cats older than 5 years

    C. Effectively transmits light and the image to the retina

        1. Very slow, even, progressive change, which may provide a clue for aging the patient

        2. When the lens precludes fundus examination, a cataract may be present

III. Cataracts—any opacity, regardless of size, of the lens or capsule (Table 12-1)

TABLE 12-1. CATARACT: PREDISPOSED BREEDS

Breed	Mode of Inheritance		Age of Onset	Position	Rate of Progression
Afghan hound	R	(?)	6 mo–3 yrs	Equatorial cortex	Progressive
Beagle	ID	(?)	Congenital	Nuclear and cortical	Progressive
Boston terrier	R	(?)	2 mo–5 yrs	Posterior cortical	Progressive
Cavalier King Charles spaniel	R	(?)	Congenital	Nuclear—± posterior lenticonus	Progressive
Chesapeake Bay retriever	ID	(?)	6 mo–6 yrs	Postaxial and equatorial cortical; nuclear	Variable
Cocker spaniel					
American	R	(?)	Any age	Posterior cortical	Variable
English		(?)	Any age	Posterior cortical	Variable
English springer spaniel		(?)	1–2½ yrs	Posterior coritcal△	Nonprogressive Slowly progressive
German shepherd	D		Aged	Nuclear and cortical	Slowly progressive
Golden retriever	ID	(?)	6 mo–3 yrs	Posterior cortical△	Stable or slowly progressive
Irish setter		(?)	Congenital–6 yrs	Posterior cortical and nuclear	Slowly progressive
Labrador retriever		(?)	1–7 yrs	Posterior cortical△	Stable or slowly progressive
Miniature schnauzer	R		Congenital	Posterior cortical and nuclear	Progressive
Old English sheepdog	R	(?)	Congenital	Cortical and nuclear	Progressive
Poodle, miniature	R	(?)	Congenital	Nuclear	Nonprogressive
Poodle, miniature and toy		(?)	3–7 yrs	Cortical—striate and clefts	Progressive
Poodle, standard	R		Congenital	Cortical— equatorial	Slowly progressive
Sealyham terrier	R	(?)	?	Nuclear and cortical	?
Siberian husky	R	(?)	1–2 yrs	Posterior cortical discoid	?
Staffordshire bull terrier	R		1 yr	Sutural flecks	?
Welsh corgi		(?)	6 mo–3 yrs	Equatorial cortical	Slowly progressive
Welsh springer spaniel	R	(?)	Congenital	Cortical	Progressive
West Highland white terrier	R	(?)	<1 yr	Posterior suture or complete	Variable
Wire-haired terrier	R	(?)	1–6 yrs	Cortical	Progressive

A. Cataractogenesis
  1. Changes in lens substance—limited to necrosis, liquefaction, fluid imbibition, and alteration of lens fiber proteins—cortical and/or nuclear, regardless of cause
    a) Initial change—cleft formation
      (1) Accumulation of products of a depressed or altered metabolism, forming clefts—diffuse watery or eosinophilic material
      (2) Probably representing altered or denatured cell proteins
    b) Cell fragments—pieces of broken lens cortical cells
      (1) Represent coagulation of protein
      (2) Cortical fragmentation or liquefaction of the cytoplasm results in the production of small or large fragments of cortical cells (Morgagni's globules)
    c) Increases in Morgagni's globules and denatured protein
      (1) Lens becomes hyperosmolar and imbibes water
      (2) Lens become "intumescent" and swollen
    d) Continual liquefaction
      (1) Results in loss of fluid through the intact capsule if the fluid is of sufficiently small molecular size
      (2) Lens becomes smaller and capsule wrinkles
  2. Changes in capsule
    a) Fibrosis anterior and posterior
    b) Proliferation of the anterior capsular epithelium
  3. Metabolic changes—Diabetes mellitus (see Suggested Readings)
    a) Glucose, galactose, and xylose (monosaccharides) all contribute to metabolism of the lens, with glucose the most important.
    b) All three monosaccharides rapidly pass from blood to aqueous.
    c) Monosaccharides are freely permeable to lens capsule.
    d) Glucose 6 phosphatase (Embden–Meyerhof pathway) has a maximum level, which is depleted when glucose level is high.
    e) Aldose reductase is in abundance within the lens and converts the monosaccharides to sorbitol, dulcitol, and xylitol, respectively.
    f) These sugar alcohols (polyols) are not permeable to the lens capsule and result in a hyperosmolar effect.
    g) Swelling (intumescence) occurs and a rapidly occurring opacity results; this may be reversible if the lens fibers don't rupture.
    h) Lens fiber rupture results, if it continues, in protein changes that cause irreversible opacity.
B. Stage of progression
  1. Incipient—water clefts and globules
  2. Immature—some clear cortex—lens may or may not be swollen
  3. Mature—swollen (intumescent) lens without any clear cortex

    4. Hypermature—loss of fluid, resulting in shrunken lens with a wrinkled capsule or liquified cortex and "sinking" of the nucleus (Morgagnian cataract)

    5. Resorption—probably associated with a tear or defect in the lens capsule that results in resorption

C. Classification—not universally accepted

    1. Chronologic—according to age—may be acquired or inherited

      a) Congenital—pre- or immediately postnatal

      b) Juvenile—occurs in a young animal

      c) Senile—5 years old or older—age is not definitive

    2. Anatomic structure and location

      a) Structure

        (1) Capsular

        (2) Cortical

        (3) Nuclear

      b) Location

        (1) Anterior

        (2) Posterior

        (3) Equatorial

        (4) Polar

D. Etiologies

    1. Acquired

      a) Inflammation—local

      b) Trauma, including surgery

      c) Radiation

      d) Diabetic

      e) Toxic

      f) Medication—shock levels of steroids cause transient posterior cortical suture cataracts in cats—may potentiate cataract formation in chronic steroid therapy in dogs

      g) Electric

      h) Nutritional—milk replacement in orphaned puppies has produced cataracts

    2. Hereditary—There are few breeds in which the mode of inheritance has been defined by breeding tests. Evidence dictates that affected dogs in a breed with a frequent incidence should not be used for breeding stock (see Table 12-1).

E. Clinical signs

    1. Signs depend on the stage of progression

      a) Incipient—subtle, small opacities anywhere within the lens or on its capsule require indirect illumination or biomicroscopic examination

      b) Immature

        (1) More distinct opacities, usually cortical, that may be observed with a pen light

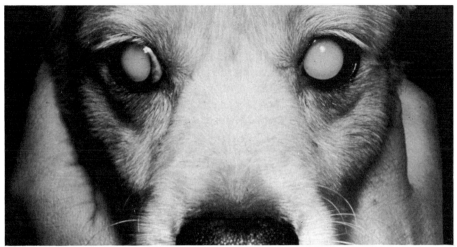

Fig. 12-3. Mature cataracts, both eyes.

        (2) Fundus is ophthalmoscopically visible
    c) Mature—usually leukocoria
        (1) Client presents animal because of visual impairment
        (2) Anterior chamber depth decreased due to swollen lens
        (3) Fundus not visible (Fig. 12-3)
    d) Hypermature
        (1) Leukocoria
        (2) Blindness
        (3) Deep anterior chamber
        (4) Wrinkled anterior lens capsule
        (5) May begin to see fundus through clearing peripheral margin
  2. Anterior uveitis—due to leakage of cataractous lens protein
    a) Normal lens protein is well tolerated by the eye
    b) Cataractous lens protein is "foreign protein" and extremely irritative to the anterior segment
  3. Change in behavior
    a) Less active
    b) Irritable
    c) Bumping into things in a familiar environment
  4. May be unilateral or bilateral
  5. Early lesions may predispose to decreased vision in bright light because of pupillary constriction
F. Diagnosis
  1. Clinical signs
  2. History
G. Treatment
  1. Medical therapy

a) Essentially, there is no effective medical therapy.
b) Mydriasis may improve vision if the opacity is axial (nuclear).
c) Diabetic cataracts—during the rapid imbibition of water and prior to alteration of the lens protein, control of blood glucose may result in clearing, but this is rare.
2. Surgical therapy
a) Unless he or she is experienced, operation is not recommended for the general practitioner; the patient should be referred.
b) Patient selection
(1) Clinical evaluation of retina
i) Ophthalmoscopic examination, if possible
ii) History of nyctalopia (i.e., signs of PRA)
iii) ERG
(2) Physical and laboratory examinations
i) Hemogram
ii) Cardiovascular evaluation
iii) Renal evaluation—BUN, creatinine, urinalysis
iv) Blood glucose—eliminate diabetes mellitus
(3) Uncomplicated cataracts resulting in blindness—candidate for elective surgery
(4) Exceptions to elective extraction
i) Anterior luxated lenses
ii) Intumescent lens
iii) Owner demand
(5) The animal must be tractible.
H. Prognosis
1. The animal will adapt to blindness without surgery.
2. Results of surgery vary—my results are about 85% successful.
IV. Lens luxation/subluxation (see Fig. 10-2 and Table 4-1)
A. Definition
1. Luxation—complete displacement from the hyaloid fossa and absence of zonular attachments
2. Subluxation—partial displacement with some zonular attachments
B. Etiologies—primary or secondary
1. Congenital/hereditary
a) Multiple ocular anomalies
b) Mesodermal dysgenesis
(1) Results in weakened or absent zonules
(2) Breed predisposition
i) Cairn terriers
ii) Manchester terrier
iii) Miniature schnauzer
iv) Sealyham
v) Wire-haired terrier
2. Trauma

3. Secondary to an enlarged (buphthalmic) eye
C. Clinical signs
   1. Iridodonesis
   2. Aphakic crescent
   3. Anterior chamber
      a) Posterior luxation—deep chamber
      b) Anterior luxation—lens visible, chamber usually deep but pupil may be obstructed
      c) Anterior displacement with iris forward—shallow anterior chamber—may be an intumescent lens
   4. Glaucoma
      a) Controversial subject
      b) I believe an uncomplicated posterior lens displacement does not predispose to glaucoma.
      c) Anterior displacement may predispose to glaucoma and should be removed.
      d) Corneal disease
         (1) Endothelial injury—corneal edema
         (2) Secondary keratopathy
D. Diagnosis—clinical signs
E. Treatment
   1. Anterior displacement—lens extraction
   2. Posterior displacement—none
   3. Concommitant disease must be treated accordingly
F. Prognosis
   1. Uncomplicated posterior displacement—good
   2. Complicated—poor

THE VITREOUS

Anatomy and Physiology

The vitreous develops in three stages, forming the primary, secondary, and tertiary vitreous. The primary vitreous develops between the lens placode and inner surface of the optic cup. It is thought that these two ectodermal surfaces contribute to the fibrillar development of the primary vitreous. Mesodermal cells migrate through the optic fissure and form the hyaloid vessel in the center of the primary vitreous. As growth and development continue, remnants of this structure persist. The anterior portion, called "Mittendorf's dot," can be seen in the adult eye on the anterior hyaloid face. The posterior aspect, called "Bergmeister's papilla," is observed rarely in dogs and cats. The space between these structures is called "Cloquet's canal." The anterior region of the entire primary vitreous is funnel-shaped and persists in the adult as the ligamentum capsulohyaloideus.

The secondary vitreous is secreted by the inner limiting membrane or foot plates of the Müller cells of the retina. As the secondary vitreous is produced, it surrounds the primary vitreous.

The third, or tertiary, vitreous differentiates into lenticular zonules (fibers) and is secreted by the neural ectoderm of the ciliary region.

The vitreous body is the largest structure within the eye, constituting 75% of ocular volume. It is transparent, containing 99% water with a collagen fiber skeleton containing a few cells (hyalocytes) whose function is unknown. The 1% solids are principally mucopolysaccharides. Hyaluronic acid, the principle component, provides the viscosity of the vitreous body. The vitreous is avascular, without nerves or lymphatics.

The vitreal attachments include the zonules, the ligamentum capsulohyaloideus, mid pars plana, and peripapillar. The anterior surface has a concavity confirming to the posterior convexity of the lens, called the patellar fossa.

Diseases

I. Congenital/hereditary diseases
   A. Normal remnants
      1. Mittendorf's dot—a spot on the anterior hyaloid membrane
         a) Approximately in the axial portion of the patellar fossa
         b) Continues posteriorly as Cloquet's canal
         c) Common in young puppies and kittens
      2. Young puppies and kittens often have degenerative remnants of the hyaloid that may be blood-filled; some have vitreal hemorrhage of no consequence.
      3. A prominent posterior remnant (Bergmeister's papilla).
   B. Persistent hyperplastic primary vitreous (PHPV) (Fig. 12-4 and see Table 4-1)
      1. In humans, PHPV is a proliferative neuroglial disease.
      2. In dogs and cats, PHPV is a persistence of the anterior hyaloid system with vascular arborization still present.
      3. Etiology—hereditary
         a) Described in Doberman pinschers as dominant with incomplete penetrance
         b) Unknown in others
      4. Breed predisposition
         a) Doberman pinschers
         b) Miniature schnauzers
         c) Beagle
         d) Others, sporadically
      5. Clinical signs
         a) Vascular network observed on anterior hyaloid face or posterior lens capsule

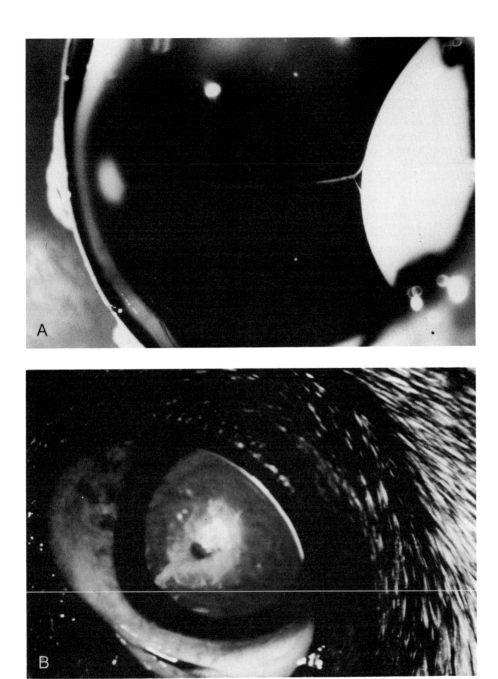

Fig. 12-4. (A) Young beagle with a persistent hyaloid. (B) Persistent hyperplastic primary vitreous in an 18-month-old miniature schnauzer. The lesion involves the posterior axial lens capsule extending into the cortex. This would not be a good candidate for an extracapsular lens extraction.

　　　　　b) Secondary cataracts
　　　　　c) Blindness
　　　6. Diagnosis—by observation
　　　7. Treatment—none
　　　8. Prognosis—good to grave
II. Vitreal hemorrhage
　A. Common in very young animals in all breeds as a congenital lesion
　B. Secondary to:
　　　1. Systemic disease
　　　2. Coagulopathy, regardless of cause
　　　3. Retinitis
　　　4. Hypertension
　C. Clinical signs
　　　1. Frequently asymptomatic
　　　2. Observed with indirect illumination
　　　3. Observe hemorrhage within or external to the hyaloid structures by ophthalmoscopy
　　　4. Severe lesions may predispose to blindness
　D. Diagnosis—by observation
　E. Treatment
　　　1. None for congenital disease—usually self-limiting
　　　2. Secondary hemorrhage—primary disease must be identified and specific therapy instituted
　F. Prognosis
　　　1. Primary disease—excellent
　　　2. Varies depending on exciting disease
III. Vitreal strands
　A. Etiologies
　　　1. Trauma
　　　2. Surgery
　　　3. Sequella to
　　　　a) Hemorrhage
　　　　b) Inflammation
　B. Clinical signs
　　　1. Gray-white fibers or cloudy masses in vitreous
　　　2. Moves or "floats" in vitreous
　　　3. Often extends from the retina to the lens
　　　4. May predispose to cataracts
　　　5. May cause retinal detachment
　C. Diagnosis—by observation
　D. Treatment—none
　E. Prognosis—depends on cause and extent of damage
IV. Asteroid hyalosis (Fig. 12-5)
　A. Degenerative hyaloid lesion observed most often in older dogs
　　　1. Unilateral or bilateral

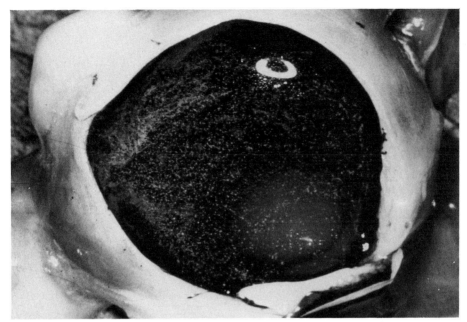

Fig. 12-5. Research miniature schnauzer with congenital cataracts and asteriod hyalosis.

      2. May be associated with previous inflammatory retinal disease

      3. Calcium lipid complexes

   B. Clinical signs

      1. Numerous refractile bodies suspended in the vitreous

      2. No clinical visual impairment—may be severe enough to compromise ophthalmoscopic examination

      3. May be observed by indirect illumination

   C. Diagnosis—by observation

   D. Treatment—none, the structures will persist

   E. Prognosis—excellent

V. Synchysis scintillans/syneresis

   A. Liquified vitreous with cholesterol precipitates that settle to the dependent part of the globe

   B. Less common in animals than in humans

   C. Clinical signs

      1. Fluid vitreous

      2. Particles can be resuspended by shaking the patient's head

      3. Often, severe lesions of the retina

      4. Often, blindness

   D. Diagnosis—by observation

   E. Treatment—none

   F. Prognosis—poor

VI. Hyalitis—inflammation
   A. Usually associated with retinochoroiditis or chorioretinitis
   B. Clinical signs
      1. Minor haze
      2. Severe purulent exudate
      3. Signs associated with primary diseases
   C. Diagnosis—by observation
   D. Treatment—primary disease must be identified and treated specifically
   E. Prognosis—varies depending on exciting disease
VII. Neoplasms
   A. No primary neoplasms
   B. Neoplasms of the perivitreal structures may involve the vitreous by extention

SUGGESTED READINGS

Blogg JR: The Eye in Veterinary Practice Vol. 1. 1st. Ed. WB Saunders, Philadelphia, 1980

Kinoshita JH: Pathways of glucose metabolism in the lens. Invest Ophthalmol 4:619, 1965

Severin GA: Veterinary Ophthalmology Notes 2nd. Ed. Fort Collins, Colorado, 1976

Appendix

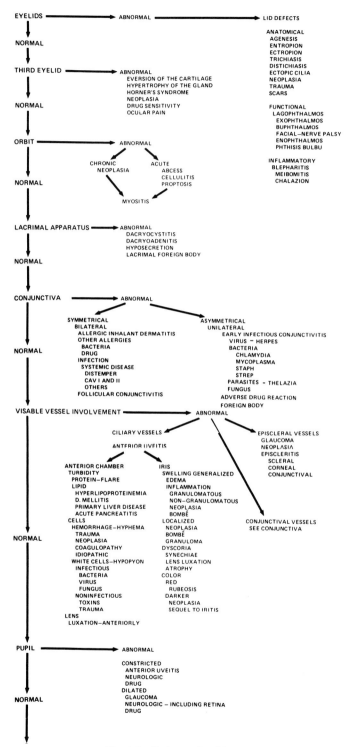

Fig. A-1. Red eye algorithm.

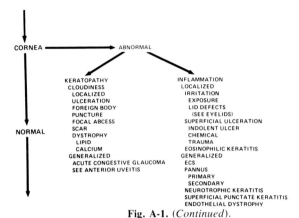

Fig. A-1. (*Continued*).

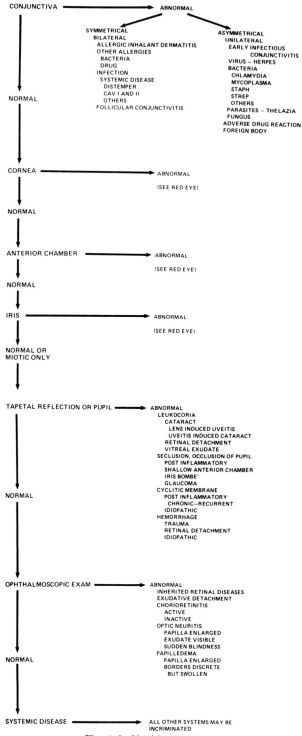

CONJUNCTIVA ────────────────────────────► ABNORMAL

                                  SYMMETRICAL   ASYMMETRICAL

SYMMETRICAL
- BILATERAL
  - ALLERGIC INHALANT DERMATITIS
  - OTHER ALLERGIES
  - BACTERIA
  - DRUG
  - INFECTION
    - SYSTEMIC DISEASE
    - DISTEMPER
    - CAV I AND II
    - OTHERS
  - FOLLICULAR CONJUNCTIVITIS

ASYMMETRICAL
- UNILATERAL
  - EARLY INFECTIOUS CONJUNCTIVITIS
- VIRUS – HERPES
- BACTERIA
  - CHLAMYDIA
  - MYCOPLASMA
  - STAPH
  - STREP
  - OTHERS
- PARASITES – THELAZIA
- FUNGUS
- ADVERSE DRUG REACTION
- FOREIGN BODY

NORMAL

CORNEA ────────────────────────────► ABNORMAL

(SEE RED EYE)

NORMAL

ANTERIOR CHAMBER ────────────────────► ABNORMAL

(SEE RED EYE)

NORMAL

IRIS ────────────────────────────────► ABNORMAL

(SEE RED EYE)

NORMAL OR
MIOTIC ONLY

TAPETAL REFLECTION OR PUPIL ──────────► ABNORMAL
- LEUKOCORIA
  - CATARACT
    - LENS INDUCED UVEITIS
    - UVEITIS INDUCED CATARACT
  - RETINAL DETACHMENT
  - VITREAL EXUDATE
- SECLUSION, OCCLUSION OF PUPIL
  - POST INFLAMMATORY
  - SHALLOW ANTERIOR CHAMBER
  - IRIS BOMBE'
  - GLAUCOMA
- CYCLITIC MEMBRANE
  - POST INFLAMMATORY
  - CHRONIC–RECURRENT
  - IDIOPATHIC
- HEMORRHAGE
  - TRAUMA
  - RETINAL DETACHMENT
  - IDIOPATHIC

NORMAL

OPHTHALMOSCOPIC EXAM ──────────────► ABNORMAL
- INHERITED RETINAL DISEASES
- EXUDATIVE DETACHMENT
- CHORIORETINITIS
  - ACTIVE
  - INACTIVE
- OPTIC NEURITIS
  - PAPILLA ENLARGED
  - EXUDATE VISIBLE
  - SUDDEN BLINDNESS
- PAPILLEDEMA
  - PAPILLA ENLARGED
  - BORDERS DISCRETE
  - BUT SWOLLEN

NORMAL

SYSTEMIC DISEASE ─────────────────────► ALL OTHER SYSTEMS MAY BE
                                                   INCRIMINATED

Fig. A-2. Uveitis algorithm.

Glossary

Abiotrophy: Trophic failure; premature degeneration or failure of vitality after reaching maturity.

Amblyopia: Reduced vision in an eye appearing normal to examination.

Amaurosis: Blindness, especially that occurring without apparent change in the eye itself.

Aniridia: Absence of the iris.

Anisocoria: The two pupils are of unequal size.

Ankyloblepharon: Adhesion of the ciliary edges of the eyelids to each other.

Anophthalmos: Total failure of the eye to develop.

Aphakia: Absence of the lens.

Aphakic Crescent: A visible crescent between the iris and lens equator due to subluxation of the lens.

Asteroid Hyalosis: Suspended vitreal calcium lipid opacities in an otherwise normal vitreous; significance unknown.

Biomicroscope (Slit Lamp): An instrument providing magnification and well-focused illumination for examination of the anterior segment and hyaloid face.

Blepharitis: Inflammation of the eyelid.

Blepharochalasis: Redundancy of the upper lid skin.

Blepharoplasty: Plastic surgery of the eyelids.

Blepharostenosis: An abnormal narrowing of the palpebral slit.

Buphthalmos: Enlargement of the eye due to glaucoma.

Canthoplasty: Surgical restoration of a defective canthus.

Canthorrhaphy: Closing the palpebral fissure at either canthus.

Canthus: The outer or inner angle between the eyelids.

Cataract: Any defect (opacity) in the transparency of the lens.

Chalazion: A cystic dilation of the meibomian (tarsal) glands, which lie in the tarsal plate; may be a chronic granulomatous inflammation.

Chemosis: Edema of the conjunctiva.

Cilium (pl. Cilia): Eyelash.

Coloboma: Any notch-like defect in the eye or lids.

Conjunctiva: The mucous membrane lining the back of the lids (palpebral) and the front of the eye (bulbar), except for the cornea.

Consensual Pupillary Reflex: Pupillary contraction resulting from light stimulation of the opposite eye.

Conus: A cone; in human ophthalmology, it refers to a myopic crescent around the optic nerve; the term has been applied to a hyperreflective ring around the optic disk of dogs and cats.

Cul-De-Sac: The fold between the conjunctival layers covering the lid and the eyeball.

Cyclitis: Inflammation of the ciliary body (pars planitis).

Cyclodialysis: Antiglaucoma operation to separate the ciliary body from the sclera.

Cycloplegia: Paralysis of the ciliary muscle, resulting in the loss of accommodation.

Cycloplegic: Drug producing cycloplegia.

Dacryoadenitis: Inflammation of the lacrimal gland.

Dacryocystitis: Inflammation of the lacrimal sac.

Dellen: A slight corneal depression due to local drying.

Descemetocele (Keratocele): Herniation of Descemet's membrane.

Diopter: The unit in which the refracting strength of a lens is designated.

Diplopia: Double vision.

Distichiasis: Two rows of cilia, with the aberrant row arising from the ducts of the meibomian (tarsal) glands.

Dysgenesis: Defective development; malformation of an organ or structure.

Dysplasia: Defective development of a specific tissue within an organ.

Dystrophy: Defective or faulty nutrition.

Ectasia: Dilation or distention; posterior, bulging away from the observer; anterior, bulging toward the observer.

Electroretinography: The recording of the changes in electric potential in the retina after light stimulation.

Emmetropia: The state of refraction of the eye in which parallel rays, when the eye is at rest, are focused exactly on the retina.

Endophthalmitis: Inflammation of the interior of the eye.

Enophthalmos: A recession of the eyeball into the orbit.

Entropion: Turning in of the lid margin.

Enucleation: Excision of the eyeball.

Epiphora: Pathologic overflow of tears.

Esotropia: Inward deviation of an eye when both eyes are opened (cross-eyed).

Evisceration: Removal of the contents of the globe with retention of the sclera.

Exenteration: Removal of all soft tissues within the bony orbit.

Exophthalmus: Protrusion of the eyeball.

Exotropia: Outward deviation of an eye when both eyes are open and uncovered.

Facet: A depression on the surface of the cornea lined with epithelium.

Fundus: The posterior portion of the eye visible with an opthalmoscope.

Gonioscopy: Study of the angle of the anterior chamber with the aid of a special contact lens and microscope or light source.

Haws: Membrana nictitans.

Hemeralopia: Day blindness.

Hemianopia: Loss of approximately one half of the visual field.

Heterochromia Iridis: Difference of color in the two irides or in different parts of the same iris.

Hippus: Spasmodic, rhythmic movements of the pupil, independent of illumination.

Hordeolum: A stye, or inflammation of the hair follicle.

Hyalitis: Inflammation of the vitreous body.

Hyalosis: Vitreal degeneration.

Hydrophthalmos: Congenital glaucoma.

Hyperopia: Farsightedness.

Hypertropia: Upward deviation of the uncovered eye.

Hypopyon: A collection of pus in the anterior chamber.

Hypotony: Low introcular tension.

Intumescence: Swelling or becoming swollen, as in the lens.

Iridencleisis: Antiglaucoma operation that uses a wick of iris to keep open a scleral defect through which aqueous drains subconjunctivally.

Iridocyclitis: Inflammation of the iris and ciliary body.

Iridodonesis: Trembling of the iris with eye movement, indicating loss of lens support.

Iris Bombé: Bulging forward of the iris due to posterior synechia.

Keratitis: Corneal inflammation.

Keratoconus: Cone-shaped deformity of the cornea.

Keratomycosis: Fungal infection of the cornea.

Keratoplasty: Plastic surgery of the cornea; corneal transplant.

Lagophthalmos: Inadequate lid closure.

Lenticonus: Conic bulging of the lens, either anterior or posterior.

Leukoma: A dense white corneal scar; an adherent leukoma is a dense white corneal scar incorporating part of the iris.

Limbus: The edge of the cornea where it joins the sclera.

Megalocornea: Congenitally large cornea, which may be confused with congenital glaucoma.

Microphthalmia: Abnormally small eye.

Miosis: Contraction of the pupil.

Miotic: A medication causing the pupil to become small.

Morgagnian Cataract: A hypermature, cortically liquified cataract in which the nucleus falls ventrally.

Mydriasis: Dilation of the pupil as the effect of a drug.

Mydriatic: A medication causing pupillary dilation.

Myopia: Nearsightedness.

Nebula: A slight corneal opacity.

Nyctalopia: Night blindness.

Nystagmus: A short, rapid, involuntary oscillation of the eyeball.

Occlusion (Pupillary): Closure of the pupil by an opaque membrane.

OD: Right eye.

Ophthalmoplegia: Paralysis of the eye muscles; Externa: Paralysis of the extrinsic muscles; Interna: Paralysis of the intrinsic muscles; Total (complete): Paralysis of both extrinsic and intrinsic muscles of the eye.

OS: Left eye.

OU: Both eyes.

Pannus: Subepithelial cellular proliferation, vascularization, and accompanying pigmentation of the cornea.

Panophthalmitis: Inflammation of all of the structures or tissues of the eye.

Papilla: A round-white disk in the fundus medial to the posterior pole of the eye; the optic disk.

Papilledema: Edema of the optic papilla (disk).

Papillitis: Inflammation of the optic papilla (disk).

Photophobia: Abnormal intolerance to light.

Photopic: Pertaining to vision in light.

Phthisis Bulbi: Shrinking of the eyeball; small, shrunken eye, following inflammation.

Polycoria: More than one pupil in an eye.

Presbyopia: Farsightedness due to loss of accommodation with old age.

Ptosis: Drooping of the upper lid.

Pupillary Block: Complete obstruction of the pupil between the posterior and anterior chambers.

Retinoscope: An instrument for the objective determination of refractive error.

Rubeosis Irides: Abnormal vascularization of the iris, usually associated with granulomatus inflammation.

Scotoma: An area of visual loss.

Scotopic: Pertaining to vision in the dark.

Seclusion of the Pupil: Annular posterior synechia.

Staphyloma: A bulging defect of cornea or sclera that is lined with uveal tissue.

Strabismus: Cross-eyed; constant lack of parallelism of the visual axes of the eyes.

Symblepharon: Adhesion of lid and conjunctiva to the eyeball.

Synchysis Scintillans: Cholesterol or fatty acids floating in a fluid vitreous.

Synechia: An adhesion of the iris to the lens or cornea.

Tarsorrhaphy: Suturing the lids together.

Tenon's Capsule: A connective tissue sheath encircling the eyeball posteriorly.

Tonometry: Measurement of intraocular pressure in mmHg.

Trichiasis: Aberrant lashes that turn against the cornea.

Vibrissae: Stiff tactile hairs around the face of animals.

Xerophthalmia: Conjunctivitis with atrophy and drying, predisposing to a dry and lusterless cornea.

Index

Page numbers followed by t represent tables; those followed by f represent figures.